TRAIN WITH INTELLIGENCE

Train Like a Champ

Harnessing Peak Performance

Dr. Cate Coker

Published by *Train With Intelligence*

United States

ISBN-13: 978-1-7353442-1-8

CONTENTS

*This book is dedicated to all those that pursue develop-
ment, growth and greater life. May the disciplines of training
reach far beyond the physical and enrich every area of your
life!*

- Dr. Cate

INTRODUCTION

V ISION. In catching the vision for this project, what came to mind was an intermingling mix of writing language that embodied leadership principles, allegory, metaphorical language, and straightforward instruction.

Why leadership principles? Leadership casts vision. It clears a path, intimately identifying with those stepping onto it. It helps readers feel understood, truly seen and hopefully impacted. Leadership takes people along a path to a finish line. Vision comes first. It is the target for direction, defining the finish line, the purpose and the mission of a journey. With that long range view in mind, the path from where we are now to where we are going, to that finish line, begins to take a trajectory. Point now to point then, here to there, it becomes clear which direction the journey takes. Defining that path requires that obstacles are evaluated, seen and deeply considered. Planning to overcome obstacles by first identifying them, then brainstorming the myriad of solutions and deciding on the most effective resolution, the results of which empower the transcendence of those very obstacles. With the journey marked out, what remains? The only thing that remains is to stay the course. Perhaps there are minor adjustments along the way. Yet, the emergence of the champ moves through the finish line with excellence and inner development like none other. The process prepared a champ. A champ from the inside out. The finish line being the expression of an inward development.

What does skillful leadership do? It builds a therapeutic relationship. Therapeutic Relating. What is that? Restoring the champ within. Recovering the original design. Moving from base-line and into prosperity of health and into peak performance. The whole person, integrated and strong. Crossing that finish line is more than the trophy, more than the accolade. The real reward is what has been built within. The substance of an athlete is worth the training.

Why allegory and metaphorical language? This language places the reader in the shoes of the champion. Step into that reality. Embody your intelligent design. Feel and see the ways your athletic systems are designed to flourish. Experience it for yourself as you read. It is in you. Let the vision seep deep into the belief of your soul and mind. How else does a champion ride out but in confidence and strength?

Create culture. How will you feel after reading this book? Empowered. Passionate. Confident. Capable. Resolute. Focused. Centered. Grounded. Self-controlled. Harnessed. Mature. Developed. Allegory builds experiential relating between concepts and the learner. It creates culture. Experiences develop working memories and affect the limbic system. An interplay between the cognitive and emotion brain, integrated learning takes root. Allegory engages the imaginative senses and draws the brain deeper into the instructional experience, blending the culture with the competence of a champion.

Straightforward instruction connects the experience and culture with concepts. Competence is the other half of excellence. It's not only what you know, it's also who you know. This rings true with the intelligent design of our brains. Not only must we be surrounded with belief and confidence in ourselves and belief and confidence from those surrounding us, but we must also have the instruction to get us where we need to go.

That is how we cross the finish line. It takes competence and culture, confidence and instruction, belief and expertise.

CHAPTER HIGHLIGHTS

Chapter 1: Creating a compelling introduction and developing the need for intelligent training, peak performance is defined. Using vision - casting leadership concepts and speaking that language to impact the heart, drawing the reader into the activated desire for peak performance training, this chapter is designed to call out the champion within you. Casting vision: What are you? The champ whispers silently, "I am the impact", "I am the prevailing force".

Chapter 2: Allegorical instruction of how peak performance plays out in the body. Giving the reader an experience, imaginative visualization is used to build understanding. Creating moments of standing in the shoes and identifying with the champ to identify and call out the champ within you. In building the context of peak performance, this chapter is designed to create personal impact and empower the vision of peak performance in you.

Chapter 3: Resonance. The impact of training, the training effect, creates resonance. Resonance is the champ, finely tuned and built from within. Developing the path of intelligent training, progressing on a journey forward, systems integration and its connection to sport is defined. Topics that build competence in training principle are as follows - Metabolic training. Central and peripheral training. Adaptation. Work Energy Theorem and its relation to kinetic energy. Kinetic Energy and the interactive sport engagement - the power of impact.

Chapter 4: Impact. The brain impacts and is impacted. Power encounter. Sport interaction. The champ is powerful, a force to be reckoned with. That force starts in the brain. Exploring the complexities of the brain and its involvement with training, this chapter highlights the following - Emotion/Cognitive Brain integration, Sensory Processing, Neuromuscular Movement, Balance, Motor Planning, Hormonal Control. Finally, how the brain toggles the switch of the autonomic nervous system (ANS) is discussed.

Chapter 5: Relating the two faces of the ANS to training and recovery, this chapter serves to explore further how the toggling of these two systems trickle into the body and respond. Allegorical picture of the champ ebbing and flowing between both is developed while also identifying rhythms that flow with these two faces. Those rhythms are as follows - Influence of hormones and brain on the ANS. Release of kinetic energy and impact with the SNS impact. Restoration of energy and building with the PNS processing.

Chapter 6: The enemy of peak performance has two faces: over and under-conditioning. Over-conditioning leads to wear and tear injuries and an overactive SNS, leading to excessive stress hormone release. Under-conditioning leads to an under active SNS, leading to reduced ability to face and overcome challenges, and ultimately, de-conditioning. Allegorical picture of the gin and yank effect of this enemy is developed as follows - Negative Adaptation. Stress Hormones in Excess. Disease and Dysfunction. Missing the Mark.

Chapter 7: Emotion brain power - the driver and influencer of the SNS/PNS activation. The balancer that keeps the yin and yang in harmony and avoids the gin and yank dissonance associated with over and under training. Harnessing its power to drive peak performance. Allegorical picture of the soul's harnessing power is developed as follows - Noble Motivations of a Champ. Limbic Lock. The Lift of Facing Truth in Training Gaps.

Chapter 8: Practical Tips to Attune Peak Performance. 13 tips to summarize and apply the intelligence of our body's design discussed in this book. The main take-away's developed and concisely reviewed for practical application. Developing the allegorical launch of the champ within, integrating the previous principles discussed.

Chapter 9: Allegorical picture of the emerging champ, fully integrated is developed. Systems integration. The power of integration versus disintegration. Finish line. Victory lap. Full circle. Champ ignited. Well done. The reward within can never be stolen. It's in you. Impacted and changed by the training. Developed.

The purpose of this book is threefold. It is to take the reader into a deeper view of the intelligence inherent in our human body; to adapt expectations, training protocol and understanding into its intelligent design; and finally, to encourage and equip the reader with an awareness of some of our body's inherent processes that are able to work and flow with peak performance training. To date, so much has been learned about the human body. It's incredible. We now have a varied and wide group of specialties in medicine and in the study of human science. More and more research develops everyday. The pursuit to continue diving deeper into the inner workings of this incredible body is a worthy and endless pursuit. So much mystery continues to surround it. It seems the deeper one dives, the more deeply one respects the complexities one finds in the dive!

I hope this book helps open the understanding of your eyes in some of what is currently known. And I look forward to the ever continuing body of knowledge that grows year by year and decade upon decade as we continue our growth and developments in the fields of human science, in all its diverse studies of the human body, and the study of medicine. The more I study the human body, the more I stand in awe of the inherent intelligence housed within it. ***Train with Intelligence*** is a project birthing to honor that design.

Thank you for joining me on this journey. Your presence completes the purpose. You are the design!

CHAPTER ONE

DEFINING PEAK PERFORMANCE

Peak Performance is the defining characteristic of intelligent training. It's a pretty important goal for all athletes. Everyone wants to hit their peak abilities when training for a sport, otherwise why train? Right. Why put the effort into a training program if the goal does not focus on attuning one's body to its peak abilities? I think we can safely say that everyone interested in a book titled, "Train Like a Champ, Harnessing Peak Performance", understands and respects the *importance* of peak performance. Yet, do we really understand what it is? Do we grasp what peak performance looks like in the human body? Do we see the complexities of our bodies and how that interplays to condition us for peak performance? Perhaps a better set of questions are these: Once we clearly identify and cast our vision for this race, do we know how to get there? What is our vision? It's the finish line. It's peak performance. What is the race? It's the path to the vision. It's the way we get to peak performance.

It's one thing to know what peak performance looks like in our bodies. Yet, it's an entirely different thing to know how to get there. Here is the premise of this book, in a nutshell. We are going to discuss both the vision and the race, the finish line and the journey. First, we will cast the vision, showing you what peak performance looks like, how it relates to you and your body as well as your sport. Then, the path to achieve peak performance will be explained. Finally, the finish line will be in your view and it will be up to you to decide if crossing that line is what you'd like to do. Let's get you over that finish line and release the inner champ within! Are you ready to emerge?

Defining peak performance, bringing our performance into a relationship with our sporting environment, and enhancing that relationship to drive an explosion of excellent and delightful athleticism is where we are going in the pages to come. Join us on this journey. Do you see the finish line? It is pure and clean athleticism.

Everyone knows pure and clean athleticism when they see it. They may not understand the depth of its mechanisms but we all recognize it, don't we? Why else do we line up at sporting events, purchase tickets, rearrange our schedules to get glimpses of the Olympic highlights, live coverages and news?

The pristine presentation of an athlete, finely tuned, causes us to stand in awe. Deep down, whether we verbalize it or not, it impacts us. The expression of human movement has the power to impact us visually, much like the expression of musical excellence has the power to impact us in an auditory manner, often becoming the music to our ears that lifts our spirits and moves us. It touches our hearts.

Excellence has the power to impact us and move us to reach further in our own lives, doesn't it? Does it not lift you and elevate your desires to stretch and grow? That is the gift of athletic excellence! Really, that is the gift of excellence. It enters sweetly into our senses, we become aware of it and we witness it. And then, excellence begins to beget further excellence. Excellence abounds from one to another in the influential complexity of community. We are impacted by one another. Reach for it. Develop. Grow. This is what our bodies were designed to do. To develop, to express, to be fruitful, multiply and progress. It's in you. Reach. Do you see your finish line? Can you visualize it, feel it? Are you hungry for it?

Like an athlete, standing at the gate, here we are. Nerves on high alert, mind strangely calm. Prepared to release the inner champ. Prepared to step onto the field and engage. Prepared to make a mark. Standing ready to produce the impact of our presence. A force, trained and conditioned. A force to be reckoned with. Powerful. Fearful. Wonderful. It's time. What are you? The champ whispers silently, "I am the impact", "I am the prevailing force". Quietly emerging, the crowd waits and watches. The champion is coming forward. Do you see it yet? Are you there? This is where we are headed. Come with me, let's reason through this together...

How does peak performance play out in the context of our lives? How does it play out in the context of our sport? One context of peak performance is that which is within our human body. It is how our body systems interact and become attuned to the efficient use of energy, the efficient expression of energy and its impact on our environment in the context of sport interaction. Another context is the reactive interplay between the athlete and the sport. It is the reaction of the sporting environment and players, the impact of our energy being rebounded back to us whether in the ground reaction forces of our surface or the contact of our opponents.

THE POWER OF ENERGY

Energy. Kinetic and potential energy. The energy of force is the kinetic energy. It is the energy that creates movement and impact. The potential energy is the training effect, where the energy is dispersed within, replenished and received, stored for the next wave of release.

The rhythm of the ocean reminds me of the rhythm of our energy systems. Ebbing and flowing. Acting and Receiving. It also reminds me of the ebb and flow in a body during training. The training stimulus is active, releases energy in the form of force, movement and impact. Kinetic energy. The release of energy from the body. Kinetic means movement. It is the defining expression of the flow of energy. It's the athlete's impact on the sporting relationship. Recovery in training is passive. It is where energy is received. Energy is replenished, used to rebuild and adapt and then stored for the next action, the next training stimulus. Potential energy. The storage of pent up energy reveals an increased potential for work. And here, we have the yin and yang of how training and recovery progressively work to condition the athlete's body, allowing it to adapt to greater expressions of the ebb and flow of energy in the sport.

It's a relating between an athlete and the interactive parts of the sport. The exchange of energy from the athlete to the sport and back again. Conditioning is the process of raising the level of that interaction to higher and higher capacities of force production. Elite athleticism is about developing force capacity in the body. It's about receiving the energy in recovery to strengthen the body to release more. Peak performance is about harnessing the development of that force exchange to hit the mark of the sport in an effort to win the prize.

High development of energy is not beneficial without a focused expression. The rhythm of our energy movements coincide with the rhythm of cognitive and emotion brain processing.

Systems integration is the mark of a peak performing athlete. Each system stands on its own and then works with the rhythm of the other systems to hit the mark, meet the goal, cross the finish line. Conditioning increases the body's ability to run the race, ride the wave, and swoosh the basketball just as the timer closes the game, the wave energy dissipates or the clock discontinues, closing a race.

There is a reactive element to sport, a relationship playing out between our impact and the response in the game. In this book, our focus is what each athlete has control over: themselves, how they act and respond in their sport. Their training regimen is their focus. It is the athlete's strategy to act and respond in their sport with intelligence. ***To train with intelligence is, to an athlete, the path to peak performance.*** What is the path? It is the journey toward our finish line, the journey into peak performance. What is the path? It is training intelligently.

Understanding the elements of intelligent training requires a study of the workings of the human body, how its systems are impacted by training. It also requires the study of the individual athlete. No two athletes are the same. The diversities are wide and so variable that applying a training regimen without a deep, intelligent study of the trainee's individuality will undoubtedly miss the mark of peak performance for that athlete. One size does not fit all just as much as one fingerprint does not define another.

The intent of this book is to bring its reader, whether an athlete, a coach, a parent, a family member, a healthcare provider or a trainer, into a deeper understanding of the human body, it's adaptation and responses to training. Then, as the vision for how peak performance impacts the human body becomes clear, the book will transition into the paths an athlete will take to cross the finish line that matches their unique fingerprint in the art and science of sport.

So what happens in the body with peak performance? Turn the page and let's see. Turn the page and let's step into the journey of a champ as she peaks in her sport.

CHAPTER TWO

WHAT'S HAPPENING IN THE BODY WITH PEAK PERFORMANCE?

P eak performance integrates and attunes all aspects of our body under one focus, one mission and one vision. It develops systems integration within the athlete. Resonating toward one vision, bringing each piece into alignment, the body focuses its energy, harnessing it toward one mission. It brings a unity to each part of the whole, even though each part is widely diverse in function and role. Unity is less about sameness and perfect conformity and more about the diverse workings operating as a unified whole. Unity is less about every cell in the body being a liver cell or a muscle cell and more about every cell in the body serving a unified purpose for the whole body. Unity is unity of purpose, unity of vision, unity of focus, unity of mission. It is a collective unity. It is a diversity of function with one vision. That vision, here in this book, for the athlete, is peak performance.

Maximizing and harmonizing our systems, priming them like a well oiled machine, is the goal of the finely tuned athlete. Each body system plays a role much like a member on a basketball team. The success of the team hinges on each member playing a part and coordinating with the whole. Coordinating well. All the same in the inner workings of the body. Peak performance requires that each system function well in their own rite and also cooperate well with other systems to bring the whole body into its vision.

Walk with me through the human body. Let's take our collective eye and tour the incredible and mysterious organization together. Let's journey on a path, stop and notice the heart, mind, lungs, energy production, energy use, strength, power, balance and flexibility of the athlete from the inside out. Let's travel together and see these things up close. What makes an athlete? What are the intrinsic and inherent operations within an athlete? We are about to see. Are you with me?

THE WARM UP

There she is. We'll start with her. Warming up at the shore line with her dynamic movements, long flowing blonde hair and her tall, long muscular frame. Anticipating the waves in her heat, mentally visualizing the elegant drop from the top of her choice wave, momentarily airborne as she descends to the surface of the curling power of water surrounding her. Visualizing the board meeting the water with an impact that her joints quietly absorb. The ripple effect of that impact coursing through the muscles of her lower legs and abdomen, her heart pounding in the rush of movement surrounding her. Working through the visual further, she imagines herself steadying her gaze forward, allowing her feet and lower body to react to the force trajectories under her board. Her arms counterbalancing the backlash against her, she lowers her body, pressing her front foot deep, preparing to press through the finish. Visualizing her triumphant finish, she presses forward, slipping through and quietly clearing the break.

Attention now turning back. Her body moving on the sand as the ocean waves roll toward her. Her muscles priming, circulation pumping as her body moves from one dynamic movement to another. Heart rate picking up slightly, autonomic nervous system shifting the body into alert action, internal heat rising slightly. Her joints, tendons and ligaments warming. Feeling the nourishment of that blood flow awakening her body, priming the internal mechanisms and waking the champ within.

It's time to rise. Becoming aware of her athletic body systems switching on, electrical impulse flowing like electricity, preparing her systems for action. It's time. Body warmed, she crouches down at the water's edge, holding her board, allowing her mind one last moment of reflection.

Settling into a state of stillness and silence, she quietly reflects on the visual screenplay that was just occupying her mind. Thinking of the breakthrough, recalling the triumphant ride out of the wave. Tasting the victory, the salt in the air around her and feeling the wave calming behind her. It's as if it's real. "Let it be", she thinks to herself. Seeing the vision of her breakthrough in her mind's eye, she whispers, "I am ready. I am ready to run after the vision". "It's time".

Coming up from her crouched position in the sand and allowing her forethought to rest steadily in the footprints that will soon be behind her, she rises and moves into the water. "Let's make this a reality", she whispers. Game on.

Her mental warm up over, her body warmed and primed, the thinking and emotion brain have unified, replaying the sequence of events, giving her a taste of what is to come and preparing her psychologically to engage the powerful, pumping energy in the surf. Diving forward, board situated under her, she paddles out. Arm moving, core compensating to sustain her balance on the board in the lack of a counter pull. Bethany Hamilton has started her heat. Or, at least this is how I imagine her starting her heat. I'd have to ask her to get the inside and concrete deets. Perhaps one day, I will.

THE POWER OF VISUALIZATION

The power of visualization takes hold of a mind being primed for performance. We see this at the start of her warm up. Why is visualization key to the warm up? What is its purpose? Visualization is the process of focusing the mind, harnessing its energy on the sport, and preparing it to perform in the direction the training prepared it for. It is engaging the power of imagination to electrically light up the central nervous system in much the same way it will light up when engaging in the sporting element. For her, that is when she is dropping in to the center of a raging barrel and moving out of it with impeccable grace and power. She is mentally living out the reality she wants her mind to create in the moments to come. With deep respect to the power of her cognitive and emotional brain processing, she is warming up the power of her decision-making as she also warms up the rest of her body.

Visualization integrates both her thinking and feeling brain. It prepares her body, processing her movements as well as experiencing how the sport engagement will feel as she acts on it with the force of her athletic presence. The visual imagery, developing in her mind, is the warm up and mental rehearsal of her peak abilities, playing out in front of her eyes. She, the number one fan. Watching, anticipating, acting, engaging. It is the expression of strength and vitality, the emotional feel and the cognitive sequencing coursing through the imaginative visualization. It is the culmination of training. Her body acting out its motor memory, releasing the vision of her peak capabilities, strengthening her belief, her drive to act and engage. Her confidence becoming firm. The screenplay of her successful vision formed. With it right before her eyes, she steps out and follows, the many times over, beaten path to the finish line of that vision. It is the familiar path of continuous and progressive training that has now become more automatic, more efficient, more effortless. It's truly a part of her now. No more intense focus. Now, simply a rhythm, a graceful movement of automaticity from a body conditioned and trained. Truly, one with her sport. Complete integration from the inside out. Finely tuned. The culminating moment. The champ within. Ready. Primed.

Why is visualization key for athletes? What is the purpose of imagining one's actions in their sport? Just as much as our physical body needs training, our brain needs training as well. Visualization trains the aspect of our brain that facilitates confidence and decisive action. Have you ever noticed how different your decisions are when you do not feel confident? How we feel about ourselves and our abilities will impact our decisions. Have you ever seen a champ cower in self doubt? Have you ever seen a powerful athlete with an expression of incapability? An expression lacking in confidence? It doesn't make sense. An expression of victory is declaring "I have overcome". It is the prevailing force against a challenge and that force is driven by the belief that one is able to prevail. That is confidence. The power of belief in one's abilities influences the ability to make the victory happen.

Confidence, how we feel about ourselves and our abilities to face challenges, is part of our emotion brain. Decision-making, what we do with how we feel, what we sense in our environment and how we'd like to act on that, is part of our thinking brain. Practicing visualization, as part of a training regimen, trains the brain to engage and rise to the challenge. It harnesses the energy of both the emotion brain and cognitive brain to work for peak performance. It lays down neurological pathways in the brain and builds habits which produce the vision of peak performance. It is part of the path to peak performance. It is intelligent training.

So, what are the keys to peak performance in these two aspects of our brain? What exactly do they do and how do they relate to training and sport engagement? Let's start with the thinking, cognitive brain. Then, we'll transition into our emotion brain. Both are required for peak performance. Both influence one another. ***Without competence, belief gets an athlete no where. Without belief, competence lacks the victorious, confident and overcoming power that ignites a champ and moves them to act.***

THE THINKING, COGNITIVE BRAIN

The thinking, cognitive part of our brain deliberates, creates and orders actions. Particularly, in the athlete, it orders the sequence of movements. It is the place executive decisions are made, including the what, where, and when of our actions.

This is where we engage in analysis, deduction, induction and comparison. It is the seat of our reasoning, logic and deliberation. Taking in information from our surroundings through our engaged senses, gathering how we feel through those senses as well as attaching meaning to that feeling in the emotion brain, our cognitive brain organizes all of this information in higher brain processing areas. In the higher brain processing centers, meaning is assigned to those senses and an action is carried out in the context of that meaning through decisive response. Calculations are made and execution of actions proceed from our thinking brain. Here, the force of our athletic presence engages the sport in response. The cognitive brain is the incubator of what the world feels like, it receives the conclusions of the emotion brain in what that feel means to the body, and integrates that data as it decides to respond and engage with its action.

In the warm up phase above, we see her moving in cognitive thinking as she decides her mental and physical warm up have concluded and her body is primed and ready to begin her paddle out. Cognitive functioning occurs as she makes snap decisions such as choosing which wave to engage and as she prepares her body to advance along its edge. It's the quick and skilled decision to respond at the right time for the desired result. It's also the skilled decision of waiting for the right opportunity to engage. It is the discipline of decisively acting as well as decisively waiting. It is knowing when to do which. Without this ability, the skillset of her actions would have no direction or focus, no self-directed navigation, no possession of self control, no harnessing power.

The executive action of the thinking brain is the director of the body. Without it, the body doesn't go. ***In athletics, it's deciding to act when the act is crucial to peak performance.*** One delay, one presumptive move, one miscalculation and an opportunity is missed. It is the power of decision-making and strategic decisive action played out on the interplay of sport. Having all the power and all the strength in the world means very little unless it is coupled with the ability to harness that power when it is most crucial. This is the power of executive cognition.

THE FEELING, EMOTION BRAIN

The counterpart to the cognitive brain is the feeling, emotion brain. When we talk about things being heartfelt and reach for the heart in our chest, that is actually a subtle misrepresentation. The heart emotions occur in our emotion brain, not at our physical heart. The emotion brain lies deep in the center of the brain and is the part of the brain that creates the emotional intelligence and culture driving our actions and decisions. It is the feel we create in our activity. It is the tone in our words. It is the meaning and value we add or subtract from our actions. It is the "how" and "why" of what we are doing. What moves you? What motivates you? Are you moved by intellect? Or, are you moved by a stirring of emotion deep within?

Excellence stirs something deep within.   Beauty stirs something deep within.   Integrated sound stirs something deep within.   We take in our environment through our eyes, ears, nose, taste and touch.   Our world "feels" a certain way to us. And sure, we can respond like a robot.   But, we don't.   We have more to our brain than the logic and technical aspect.   We have an emotion brain that creates the emotional tone of our expressions.   We are moved and motivated by meaning.   It is the assigning of meaning that causes us to take action.   What is meaningful to us?   What has value?   Our values move us.   Values are very individual.   They are one of the aspects of our humanity that are not externally defined but internally defined.   We act out our values everyday.

Our senses not only impact our cognitive and technical functions in our thinking brain, they also impact our more qualitative and soul aspects of our emotion brain.   Our brains include both logic, reason and memory as well as emotion, tonal expression and soul.   We are both quantitative and qualitative in nature.   Quantitative measures alone would reduce us to mere robots.   Whereas a qualitative focus alone would not move us anywhere.

Did you ever notice how what moves one person may not move another?   There is a substance within each person, a predisposition to resonate with some things while an indifferent consideration for others.   What causes us to differentiate that? Is this, too, much like the unique stamp of our fingerprint?   The art behind our humanity in which no two individuals carry the same expressive identity? Perhaps this is where the personality, preferences, and temperaments play out in the diversity of humanity. The impact of our unique stamp, completely possessed by a fully activated and integrated individual. Are you resonating with your design? Is this where we are designed for a purpose with natural gifts, talents and predispositions to impact our world around us?

The emotion brain is moved by a substance within us that cannot be neatly quantized. It is not easily measurable, perhaps because it is what slips out of our bodies as we take our last breaths here. The slipping of our soul that brought a body to life. What brings you to life? What resonates with you and ignites a motivating movement within you?

The emotion brain is the seat of motivation. It is the intuitive, relational component in our thinking and decision-making. Here, we relate to ourselves in self awareness, we develop empathy and compassion for ourselves and others, we begin to understand self regulation and self control, and we learn the art of considering others as well as ourselves in our actions. It's a place of association by relationship and where we become interdependent individuals, connected securely to community and to our sense of self and unique identity.

The common phrase, "it's not what you know, it's who you know", is referring to the power of emotional intelligence housed in the emotion brain. That phrase is speaking to the intelligent ability to build personal self control, strong relationships and a community of support. That takes skill. And it's a different skill than what the cognitive brain develops. Of course, in an integrated and finely tuned athlete, it's less a choice of one or the other and more a development of both the emotion and cognitive components functioning well together. Perhaps I would rephrase it to say "It's not only what you know, it's also who you know". Put another way, having the competence in technical skill is just as important as attaining competence in emotional development. It is the integrated blend of both the emotion brain and thinking brain.

The emotion brain sees the world through the lens of relationships and associations. It associates our beliefs and feelings with our cognitive brain function. For the athlete, this aspect becomes valuable as we associate feelings with our actions. The culture we choose to saturate our minds with has a profound impact on the state of our mind, the state of our executive cognition. Negative emotional constructs like self-doubt, enmity, envy, jealousy and ill will drive our psychological culture and morale into a toxic environment. Have you ever heard the phrase "who you surround yourself with will make or break you"? If you are surrounded largely by people stuck in negative emotional constructs, it will cripple your own emotional construct. No one can reach their peak allowing the emotion brain within them to self destruct into toxic feelings and thoughts. The usefulness of what you know has the potential to be severely hampered or strongly empowered by who you know. One affects the other.

THE INTEGRATION OF EMOTION AND COGNITION

Oddly, we sometimes don't realize the importance of attuning these two brain functions to work for our vision and unfortunately they can become a source of great obstacle in our pursuit toward peak performance. Patterns of destructive emotional constructs play out in our cognitive processing, leading us toward self-destructive outward actions. In athletics, this results in an athlete that is primed and able to perform well in other systems yet unable to express that excellence because of the lack of systems integration here in the emotion brain. There's no spark, no fire, no confident motivation to carry the competence through to completion.

All cylinders are not priming in the same direction. When there are two visions, two directions, two finish lines we are aiming toward, our bodies become divided and our systems work against one another. Systems disintegration is at the helm and the beginning of an undermining break in the foundation of our abilities occurs as subtle self-defeating and self-destructive mechanisms remain unchecked and unaddressed. The importance of the emotion brain, left ignored, topples the athlete much like a three-legged table attempting to stand under the weight of a five course meal.

Attuning our minds, both the emotion brain and cognitive brain, are a crucial piece of athleticism. Toppling and crumbling of so much extraordinary capability does not need to occur. And that is the good news. It's why we are here, on this journey together, paving a clean path toward our vision. The vision of peak performance. The vision of clean and pristine athleticism.

Now that we've looked at the emotional and cognitive intellect operating in this athlete, let's talk about how the mind impacts the body. What is happening in the dynamic movements of her warm up? What role does our nervous system play in our warm up? Specifically, what role does our autonomic nervous system play? What role does the sympathetic autonomic system play in releasing the inner champ, the athletic warrior? How does it begin to wake up that sleeping giant? What activates it?

SYMPATHETIC NERVOUS SYSTEM ACTIVATION

Imaginative visualization during a warm up activates the emotion brain. It gives the body an experience to process and prepares the body to act according to that vision. With the emotion brain engaged, signals get sent to the area within the brain that activate the hormonal cascade as well as the nervous system that engages the body for action.

There is a two fold purpose in a warm up. It not only prepares the mind, both in thinking and in emotion processing, but it also turns on the sympathetic nervous system and prepares the body for engagement. There are two ways our brain, the central command center, shifts the body into a collective direction. In this case, that direction is sport engagement. Those two ways are through the nervous system and the hormonal system. Both of which are switched on by the influence of the emotion brain.

Dynamic stretching combines mobility and muscle lengthening in whole body movement patterns. It is an active warm up, allowing blood flow to heat the body internally and introduce movement gradually. The mobility in dynamic stretching serves to circulate and shunt blood flow into the further reaches of the body, into the muscles and limbs. The movement in a warm up also facilitates a gentle shift into an alert nervous system state, preparing the active body systems for work. Remember, we are impacted from our command center as well as influenced by what our body does at the periphery, meaning movement facilitates brain engagement and the brain facilitates movement.

The body has two states of being, the resting state and the active state. Behind the scenes, the body is active at all times even when we are not. Our activity depends more on voluntary operations and our rest depends more on involuntary and automatic processes that support our voluntary work. The body is either involuntarily active in operations of rest, replenishment, rebuilding and recovery or voluntarily active in force of impact and use of that replenishment. For the athlete, this correlates with training recovery and training work. These two opposing processes are supported by two nervous system operations. The parasympathetic nervous system steps to the forefront during resting mechanisms. While the sympathetic nervous system comes forward to prime the body for action.

When our body is in an active state, the predominating sympathetic nervous system, or the alert nervous system, targets body functions that harness physical movement and focus. In this state, the blood begins to shunt away from the resting state nervous system and their respective organ system functions and starts moving its resources to the muscles, the heart, the lungs and the furthest reaches of the frame, waking and preparing the champ for action.

The warm up visualization primes the body's sympathetic activation from the brain, turning the periphery on. The warm up at the periphery, in the dynamic movements, places a demand on the brain, signaling the emotion brain to stimulate the sympathetic nervous system further and release the hormonal cascade to support the body and prepare it to meet the challenge.

The body operates and responds to demands placed on it. These demands can be internal, through the executive cognitive function. We decide and then we act. At times, they can also be external, creating a real time and quick reaction. We act and then our thinking aligns and we make better decisions. The central directs the periphery and the periphery has the power to affect the central.

When the demand clearly communicates that the sympathetic nervous system is necessary, the body responds by creating this gradual shift away from resting state and into an active and ready for action state by activating the sympathetic nervous system and inhibiting the parasympathetic system. These two systems ebb and flow. They do not operate simultaneously in full strength. When one is active, the other pulls back. They stimulate opposing body states. One brings the body into action and the other brings the body into the active work of rest and recovery. Training requires both recovery and work. The autonomic nervous system is what guides these phases of training. Over or under training is linked to the loss of the delicate balance between these two aspects of the autonomic nervous system.

The body produces and shifts its balances and resources based on the demand placed on it. As the mind prepares the vision and direction of its action, the body begins alerting and preparing the demand for action through its warm up. As the body moves through the warm up, the brain is stimulated and the cycle compounds until the body is fully active. The body follows the mind, its director, and mobilizes according to the vision. The mind is influenced by the body's actions. Systems integration. This is how the mind impacts the body. And how the body impacts the mind. The sympathetic nervous system predominates, the body systems involved in producing action ignite, firing up with the electric power of our nerves. Internal organ systems not predominantly involved in engaging in the sport take a backseat and rest from their work. The systems involved step forward. Do you see the balance? Meeting the demand. The engagement of the body is remarkable. We see the power of the body's response to the challenge. Let's take a deeper look again.

THE CHAMP IGNITED, SYSTEMS ARE A GO!

As her vision focuses, the sympathetic nervous system adjusts and dilates her eyes as she deeply takes in her sporting context, the surface, and the waves forming with greater clarity. Distracting visual sights around her fall into the back seat of her mind as her eyes become primed to focus and engage. Adrenaline releases as a result of the nervous system shift. It courses through her body, elevating her heart rate and her heart's ability to press her blood further and quicker through the furthest parts of her body. Her body heat is increasing, warming the joints, tendons, ligaments and muscles. Flooding them with circulation and blood flow, clearing out stagnate cellular waste. Her muscles stretch, move easily and begin contracting more efficiently. Her breathing rate increases slightly, reaching deep into her lungs, deep into her bronchial tubes. The pathway into her lungs opening wide, with a greater flow of oxygen entering and carbon dioxide leaving. Meeting the demand. The power of adaptation.

Oxygen floods her blood stream. The speed and power of her heart contraction increasing slightly, pressing the blood even further to the muscles of her limbs. Standing at the shore, her body is primed for action. She's been here many times and intuitively knows when her sympathetic nervous system has switched her athletic systems on. She knows her body well. Her warm up complete. "I'm ready", she says as she exhales one last deep breath and steps into the ocean, board in hand.

PRIMING THE CHAMP AT THE HEART AND LUNGS

The sympathetic nervous system is on full speed now. Its impact on the heart and lungs evident in her, engaging these two organ systems to meet the demand of peak performance and elevating the work of both of them. The lungs opening to take in larger amounts of oxygen and the heart working more to spread that oxygen throughout the body. Taking oxygen to the active muscles of the body is important in producing energy to perform. Peak performance requires energy to make an impact.

IMPACT

What exactly is impact? Let's take a moment and define that. Impact is the power of an athlete's presence in the game of sport. It is the force production of the body being released into the game. Remember that energy is released and then replenished in an athlete through training and recovery. With energy release in a game, force is produced and exerted on a sporting medium and then rebounded back to the athlete. This is the interaction of sport. And sport is the interaction of energy. Energy bounding between one participant and another, one athlete and their sporting surface. How does the sympathetic nervous system prime the body to make an impact?

The sympathetic nervous system is the switch that turns on that impact in an athlete. It is the face of impact that comes to the surface in our body, the "game face" of the champ emerging. When the SNS is on, it alters and shifts actions within many body systems to prepare for impact. To prepare for the power of a forceful release. We began discussing the heart and lungs. Let's move into some details about the body systems that are impacted by the SNS, which then reverberates that impact through the body, releasing it onto our sport.

BLOOD FLOW, WHERE DOES IT GO? WHAT DOES IT DO?

The cardiorespiratory system brings together the function of our lungs, our heart and our blood vessels. In the lungs, the oxygen that we breathe in enters deep into the airways. Once the oxygen has reached into the depth of the lungs, it then shifts into the blood vessels. The blood vessels circulate the oxygen filled blood into the heart and is then pumped throughout the body by the powerful pumping mechanism of the heart muscle. Our blood vessels form an internal circuit between the cells of our body, the lungs and the heart, allowing the flow of blood to touch every part of the body when and as it is needed.

BLOOD VESSELS

Blood vessels, the internal circuit of our body, are a closed system. There are parts of the vessels whose linings become open just enough for certain substances necessary to nourish cells to pass through the lining, but the closed system is designed to maintain the blood flow within the vessels. The blood is a carrier. The smaller areas of the closed circuit help release the transported substances carried in the blood, such as oxygen. They also help substances enter the blood flow to be carried and released at different places within the body as needed. Other examples are carbon dioxide and energy in the form of blood sugar.

DRIVING THE AIR FROM THE LUNGS TO THE CELLS

The exchange of oxygen in and carbon dioxide out occur at the cellular level and is what we call cellular respiration. As the lungs are involved in respiration of these same gases, that respiration is made possible much deeper in the body at the cellular level by the intricate internal circuit and transport system of the blood.

INTERPLAY OF BREATHING, DRIVING IT DEEP

Looking at the entire circuit again, we have the lungs taking in oxygen and breathing out carbon dioxide. Within the lungs is an extension of the blood vessel circuit that leaks out carbon dioxide as it takes in oxygen. The blood flowing through that circuit is flowing toward the part of the heart that presses it into the furthest reaches of the body through the force of its muscular contraction. This section of the blood vessel circuit is called the arteries. It is the path of the blood flow from the heart to the lungs, then back in to the heart where it is then sent to the cells. Respiration thus extends from the lungs and into the cells.

On the return, the cells release carbon dioxide into the blood flow while the oxygen is consumed in the energy production process. This is the point, at the cellular level, that the blood vessel circuit becomes what we call the veins. As the blood flows back to the heart, through its closed system and circuit, it reaches the lungs. Carbon dioxide is released from it and the lungs exhale that substance back into the atmosphere, into the air we breathe. The breaths we take are driven down to the very depths of our bodies through the work of the blood. It's as though the breath reverberates through our body, from external to internal and then internal to external.

THE HEART OF IT RECAPPED

There is an important relationship between the heart, lungs and our blood circulation. All three of these work together to help build energy for athletic impact. The heart is the muscular force that propels blood, the lungs recycle the two very important gases within the blood, filling blood with new oxygen at every breath and retrieving the carbon dioxide to exhale out as we breathe. Finally, the circulation, the blood vessels that allow the blood to reach every part of the body, carry the nutrients and other substances important for energy.

From the heart and lungs and on the way to the cells, we have the arteries that carry those substances that produce energy at the cellular level. Not only is the oxygen necessary from the air we breathe in our lungs, but the nutrients that we eat become necessary as well. When the body is in active mode, the nutrients that have been processed and stored for energy are released into the blood stream. The blood carries them in the arteries to the cells. The cells take in the nutrients and oxygen, and use those products to release energy in a biochemical process called cellular metabolism.

SUSTAINING BASIC ENERGY - BASAL METABOLIC RATE

The blood needs to touch and interact with every cell in the body, from our organs sitting within our central trunk to the very extensions of our toes and fingers. The reason for this is that the blood provides the life source, the nutrients containing energy and the oxygen we breathe in, for every aspect of the body to remain alive, functional and healthy. Without adequate blood supply, cells die. For life to be maintained and for the body to stay out of a diseased state, blood flow must remain unhindered. Not only does the blood carry the life source for every cell, it also is crucial in providing energy to support greater exertion in athletic work.

This basic life support is called our basal metabolic rate. It is the base level of energy production required to sustain life in everyday activities. It sustains the life of every small component of the body, which we call "cells" in the human science language. Blood flow and the delivery of oxygen to these cells increases dramatically during exercise and is crucial to peak performance.

ENERGY SOURCES - AIR & FOOD

Energy, in our world, is conserved. Meaning, it is the impact of the world on us as much as our impact back on the world. Energy transforms from one form to another as it rebounds between us and our world. We derive our energy from foods and the air in our atmosphere. We breathe in the oxygen, we take in the food through our mouths and begin the work of digestion as it enters our digestive tract. What we take in fuels us to release energy and create impact.

Just a little neat side note: the digestive tract is actually considered to be outside of our body! It is an internal tube specialized in mechanically and chemically breaking down the energy source of our food. Food components are broken down into its smallest chemical structure. It is in these structures that energy is held. These small, energy conserved, digested and broken down components of the food we eat get taken into and absorbed in our body through the lining of our digestive tract. The food is broken down only to the extent that the energy within them remains conserved and intact. This is the point that what we eat actually enters our body! And well the food components that don't enter exit this outside, yet inside tube. It is like an internal funnel designed somewhat like a juicer as it mechanically and enzymatically disassembles food and prepares it for entrance into the body, for its use and its storage. Once inside, our body uses some of the energy for basic life support, our basal metabolism, our basic energy production. Our simple existence requires consistent energy. The remainder is stored within our body to be retrieved in work and peak performance. It is retrieved when the energy needs are greater than the basic life need.

As the SNS is activated and the body becomes active, the breathing increases causing more oxygen to enter the blood. In addition, the work of the heart increases and blood begins to circulate with greater speed throughout the body. The hormonal system activates a cascade that releases the stored energy nutrients into the blood stream. Together with the oxygen and the nutrients, the arterial blood moves toward the cells in the body, releasing its contents into them through a process called cellular respiration and other transport mechanisms. Once within the cell, cellular metabolism begins.

Cellular metabolism is the harnessing of the energy within the nutrients. Remember that digestion broke down the nutrients while keeping the energy within them intact to allow the body to absorb them, process them, use what was immediately needed and then store the remainder. Cellular metabolism continues that process to release the energy in the process of doing work! Thus, our body consumes energy in stages. Both in steadily breaking it down and containing the energy until its needed. In doing so, work is done.

THE DEPTH OF OUR BREATH

Oxygen is required to help break the nutrient down further and release its energy in a form that produces the juice behind the actions of peak performance within the cell. This is where cellular respiration meets cellular metabolism. It is where oxygen slips into the cell, or breathes into the cell. Cellular respiration. Think about it. What is respiration? It is breathing in oxygen and out carbon dioxide. While this happens at the lungs, it also happens at the cellular level. Breathing in oxygen deep within the cells, the amount of oxygen that passes through the cell is a key indicator for fitness! Building efficiency, the breath externally runs deep and supplies the internal energy production with its resource, oxygen. The more oxygen that runs deep into the cells, the more energy is produced efficiently.

Along with the hormonal cascade signaling the release of stored nutrients, there is a complicated system of conversions that release the stored energy. Those conversions and metabolic pathways only engage according to the type of activity demand

and the availability of oxygen. The inherent intelligence within our cells determines which way to produce energy. It chooses the most efficient pathway based on what is presently available in the form of energy from food sources and oxygen.

HARNESSING ENERGY FOR ATHLETIC WORK

Energy must be a form that is usable in our body and that is what cellular metabolism does. It transfers the energy into a form that our body is able to use, matching it to the type of movement and physical demand we are creating, and fueling energy to meet the demand. Our body has three systems of harnessing and releasing energy from our nutrients and into the cells to fuel our body. The specific activation of any one of those systems is dependent on an interplay between oxygen availability, nutrient availability and type of physical exertion. Those three systems are the phosphagen system, the aerobic system and the anaerobic system. Their activation is dependent on the physical exertion we place on our body. Peak performance places a demand on our metabolic systems. The various ways we express that energy release in athletics causes a shift and blending in which of these systems are put to use. For athletes, training metabolically has the power to shift the body's capacity to handle remaining within systems with increasing physical exertions. The capacity of each system can be trained and expanded in the athlete. We will get into metabolic training in more detail in the next chapter. The incredible thing about the human body is its capacity to adapt. Training requires that the body adapt to higher levels of energy production, energy expression and energy efficiency. In cellular metabolism, athletic expression is fueled. Energy is used when the need is present. Training trains the body's use of energy by strategically building an intermittent need and strengthening its production systems to work more efficiently.

The oxygen is a major player in producing energy throughout the entire body. We've touched on this some in discussing cellular respiration (how our breath enters cells) and cellular metabolism (how cells use our breathing as they build and release energy).

FULL CIRCLE OF CIRCULATION

Remember, the closed loop system of circulation runs like this: from the furthest places of our body, after blood has exhausted its oxygen supply and given it to the surrounding cells, the blood moves back toward the heart through the portion of the circulatory loop called the veins. As this blood is carried back toward the center of the body, it enters the right side of the heart. As the heart contracts, this side of the heart ejects blood into the lungs. Here, it picks up the oxygen in the lungs and lets go of the carbon dioxide it retrieved from the cells. By the way, carbon dioxide is the waste product from energy being produced in a cell and needs to be removed from the body. Do we again see the beauty of the deep internal breath of the cell releasing itself from the inside out and back into the atmosphere? Carbon dioxide released. And released again through the powerful elastic recoil of our lungs. As this exchange takes place, the blood becomes filled with oxygen again and travels to the left side of the heart where it fills the lower portion of it. The blood is then powerfully ejected back into the circulation loop with the power of the heart's contraction and muscular strength. On a quick side note, this contraction is what creates "blood pressure" and we'll get into that later. For now, let's follow the blood through the rest of the loop. As the blood is pumped back out of the heart and into the periphery of the body, it is located in the portion of the closed circulatory loop called the arteries, containing oxygen and supplying the needs of the cell. As blood travels, releasing oxygen to cells, in exchange, it picks up the waste product of carbon dioxide to be cycled out of the body in respiration. So, in recap, after the blood lets go of its oxygen and picks up carbon dioxide, it enters the right heart and then the lungs and retrieves oxygen. It then enters the left heart and is pumped out again throughout the body to fuel energy production! Pretty simple, eh? Well, it does have more complication than that but we'll build on that over time.

PLANT LIFE AND OUR LUNGS

Now, let's focus on the lungs. We breathe in atmospheric oxygen and we breathe out carbon dioxide. This makes sense now because of how our body uses both of these gases. On a neat side note, our relationship to plant life is symbiotic. As we breathe in air, we breathe in the presence and evidence of other life in our world. Meaning, our lives are deeply intertwined with the world. In just one example, as we breathe out the carbon dioxide, the plant life takes it in as its source of energy production. The exhale of their life reaches the atmosphere as it breathes out oxygen as a waste product for its systems. What is one's trash becomes another's treasure. Is there really trash? Or is energy recycled? We pick up the oxygen they breathe out and we have this very neat and complementary relationship! Just thought I'd add some plant love here. Plants nourish our air with what we need to survive. We nourish the air with what they need to survive. Destroying plant life destroys our life. I'll just leave that right there, ok. Surround yourself with plants, its good for health!

So, back to our lungs. As we inhale, the diaphragm, which sits below our lungs, draws downward and creates a negative pressure system in our lungs, creating an influx of air as the lungs expand in response to the action of the diaphragm. The deeper the inhalation and the bigger the breath taken in, the more of our lungs become filled with oxygen and the more carbon dioxide is released from the blood and back into the air as the blood routinely circulates the lungs. As the lungs recoil back to their original position, air is released out and the carbon dioxide is released out of the body into the atmosphere. The lungs are the housing mechanism of our interaction with the atmosphere. Air comes in, air goes out. Somewhat like the digestive tract. Food enters the tract, but not all of it enters the body. Entrance into the body requires entrance into the blood. The two systems that drive energy production interact with our environment to receive the material to convert that energy into the form used by our body to be energetic!

Now, the blood circulation is quick and constant. So is our breathing. With exercise, of course, both of those processes get even quicker. We know that, during exercise, our breathing rate increases as well as the circulation of our blood because of the faster heart beat and greater blood volume released with each beat. The harder we work in exercise, the more our cells need oxygen to produce energy and keep our systems going strong. This demand drives our circulation to increase, our heart to pump stronger and quicker and our breathing rate to increase to accommodate the quicker flow of blood through the lungs and maximize on the opportunity to exchange the gases of oxygen and carbon dioxide that we've been talking about. This is called ventilatory perfusion. The amount of the atmosphere that interacts, entering and exiting, our blood. On the other end is what is called maximal oxygen uptake. The blood perfusion in the opposite direction. It is oxygen pressing into the cell in cellular respiration. Why is this important? Our bodies are able to grow and adapt in their ability to take in more oxygen at the lungs and at the cells. One is called central training and the other is called peripheral training. The next chapter will touch on this further as we shift into discussing the effects of training on the body's systems. Let's get back into the game for a moment.

PADDLING OUT - PRIMED FOR ACTION

Duck diving through the white wash, she presses her arm against the board, driving it deep, below the break. Tucking her head and diving through, she returns to the surface of the water. Gliding along the surface of the water, drawing closer, the steady pumping of her arm forward increasing her breathing rate, her heart pumping to catch up to the demand, yet intermittently pausing by a quick dive under the energy release in the resounding, reverberating residual effects of the set's impacts on the ocean's surface.

METABOLIC SHIFT - PHOSPHAGEN TO AEROBIC

The increase in breathing rate and the initial spike in her heart rate as she begins her cardiorespiratory work of paddling out is indicative of the moment her body begins to adapt to the new demand of activity placed on it. The initial metabolic energy producing system used in all movement activity is the phosphagen system. The sharp change causes the body to kick into high metabolic shift. The phosphagen system takes up the slack while the elevated breathing rate and heart rate catch the body up to the oxygen demand. Once the oxygen reaches the muscle cells, the body shifts into the aerobic metabolic energy production. The heart rate normalizes and the body is on track.

COMPETITVE ZONE

She's in the competitive zone now. Her professional surfing peers nodding, with an air of deep respect for the mutual love of surf and ocean and yet, simultaneously, shooting each other that recognizable glance of competitive rivalry as they each turn to focus on the set rolling in and under them.

THE NOBLE HEART OF CHAMPIONS

The dignity of powerful champs, lining up to showcase their development. The air is electric with a sense of nobility. Excellence begets excellence and it is playing out now. The limbic system is locking and the power of influence roles out with the pumping energy of the surf. The emotion brain elevating and a surge of hormone releasing into bloodstreams. The hormonal input that rushes the body with a sense of purpose, honor and respect, adjusting body chemistry, preparing the emotion brain to peak and drive the cognitive brain into constructive action.

LIMBIC LOCK

The power of relational influence playing out. Surrounding themselves with champion hearted contenders, the competitors shift the emotional tone of the event. The feel and culture of dignity erupts. The limbic system is releasing powerful motivators with constructive emotion undergirding the abilities of the athletes. Confidence and power in the emotional atmosphere is rolling out with the power of the surf under them.

VISUAL SCAN MEETS EMOTION BRAIN

To what the eyes see and take in, the emotion brain adds meaning. Remember, we are influenced by our environment and we are the influencer of that environment. As our eyes focus on healthy emotional motivators, our emotion brain moves to influence our cognitive brain.

With the board under her, head up, she scans the water's surface. Looking at the flow of energy rolling along the surface, she quickly studies the ocean's rhythm and timing. Her eyes lock onto her destination. She sees her set powerfully rolling in. Taking a moment to think, deciding where to position herself, and patiently waiting, the excitement echoes in her and a smile begins to crack on her lips. This is it.

VISUAL SCANNING MEETS COGNITIVE BRAIN

The eyes engaged, scanning the development of the wave, her cognitive brain begins processing that visual input. The details of this sensory information quickly transmitted to her thinking brain for analysis. All of this happening in a matter of milliseconds. With the cognitive executive in her mind, calculating and directing her, the decision is made and this information is then delivered to the parts of her body that develop the response. All of this, again, happening in a matter of milliseconds. It is the power of her training in action.

Motivation set and strong. Eyes scanning and preparing the body to move. The competence of the "what", "when" and "where" undergirded by the "why" and "how". The emotion brain building the confidence to strike with competence. The integration of the emotion and cognitive brain is the connection between confidence and competence.

AUTOMATICITY - THE CULMINATION OF MOTOR LEARNING

Her body has been conditioned to respond in this sporting context. The adaptation of her training has transferred this once conscious and laborious action into an action of automaticity. The power of the athlete, finely tuned. Fully engaged.

Motor learning is the brain's automaticity training. It involves the deep brain processing centers that create habits. Habitual actions require less focus. This is where they become more automatic, allowing it to happen while engaging and focusing the body elsewhere simultaneously.

HORMONAL INFLUENCE

Smiling and at ease, her emotion brain flooding the body with hormonal stimulus and producing the enjoyment of this moment. Some anticipation, some nervous energy is normal. Yet, there is no debilitating fear. No paralyzing analysis. No emotional memories flooding and distracting her mind as she moves forward. There is peace and her mind is able to focus without being weighed down in painful and discouraging thoughts or emotions. She has all the feel goods driving her nervous anticipation, directing it into the power of her abilities. Releasing possibility, believing in her ability to overcome and stretching toward the challenge with confidence. Securely putting herself out there, taking her calculated risk, and riding this wave, knowing the wave may take her under. Yet, deciding to face the wave, make her impact and bring the best of her to the encounter. Playfully toying with the waves to come. Who knows? "Maybe the powerful energy of the wave cannot stand the power of my impact", she thinks to herself. This is the power of her emotion brain working for the vision of peak performance, her confidence resonating and reverberating within her, producing an outlook of perception that strengthens her to step into her challenge and face the fear. It's the engagement of her sport, seeing the wave less as the fearful energy force it truly is and more the synchronization of an athlete and her sport becoming more unified, more in tune. The energy rhythms of one ricocheting off the other in the elegant dance as her board meets the water's edge, preparing to showcase the skill of her athletic force along the strength of the ocean's energy wave.

THE ELEGANT DROP - THE PROPRIOCEPTIVE TOUCH

Core engaged, arm pressing deep into the water, propelling her forward, her asymmetric pull works for her. Gliding gracefully and powerfully across the water, the set begins to lift under her. It's the power of the wave, the break of its edge forming under her. The feel of the water changes, the surface becoming more chaotic. It is here. She lets the water propel her further into the chaos of the lift. Pressing through her arm, lifting her body. Driving her legs under her, she stands on the board at the edge of the break.

The feel of the board under her, the sense of her body responding to the movement of the water beneath her, she moves with an intuitive sense. Positioning her feet on the board, aware of where her body is without actively looking at it.

What is this sense? Her ability to know where her body is in relation to the water at any point in time? Proprioception. Within her joints are many sensory receptors that give her brain an internal map of what every aspect of her body is doing as it is doing it. Detailing her orientation in space, she is able to close her eyes and engage her body in many ways as if she was watching every move from the outside of it. Proprioception helps her move with balance and precision. It fine tunes the focus of her vision. Much like an internal mind map vision, she is free to engage her visual sense on her surroundings while her internal body map, her proprioceptive sense, reconciles its movement with the visual planning of what is around her.

THE ELEGANT DROP - WHERE BALANCE & VISION INTERTWINE

Slipping off the ridge, momentarily airborne, she drops into the center of the circling force of energy. Heart pounding, adrenaline rushing through her, she lands on the water's surface. Her feet reacting quickly to the forces hitting her board, body adjusting to the changing surface, her eyes focus forward. Assessing the breaking point and her estimated distance, she adjusts and drops lower, deepening the front foot to adjust her speed and stay ahead of the tunnel forming behind her.

THE ANAEROBIC SUDDEN SHIFT

Heart pounding, racing from the sudden change in movement, the sudden shifts in positioning and muscle engagement. The sudden change creating an immediate demand in energy. Her energy systems shifting with the change, moving toward the anaerobic system as her breathing and heart rate catch up and supply the oxygen needed to switch back into the more enduring aerobic energy systems. Her body keeping pace, the subtle shifts occurring as her heart rate normalizes.

THE FINISHING TOUCH - BREAKING THROUGH

Coming out through the end, the water crashing down around her, legs steady in a deep squat, holding her line under the dispersion of forces impacting the board, she emerges. Breaking through, her legs ease up.

NEUROMUSCULAR CONTROL

The power of her balance held against the impact of the wave surrounding her. The brain simultaneously taking in the adjustments at her feet, the forces coming at her board, the visual of the wave forming before her. Within milliseconds, the corrections coming through with electric speed, adjusting the fine movements of her body to remain in position as she rides the tumultuous wave through its tunnel.

THE SALTY TASTE OF SWEET VICTORY

Using her back leg to steer, she squats slightly, bending her front leg, leaning heavily on her back leg, extending it. With the weight focused on the heel of her back foot, she presses the weight of her heel down and slightly forward, spinning the back end on an upswing. Lightening up on her front foot, she ascends the remaining wake of her wave. Midway up, she pulls her front leg out of the squat some, applies a downward, stabilizing force through the ball of her foot. Her back heel whips strong in a powerful upswing. Hips ride back while her upper body and chest ride heavily forward. Arms leading the turn, slightly airborne as she skates across the lip of the wake. Front toes gripping and driving the board back into the base, her back heel and mid foot finish the turn with a downward force as the board stabilizes back into the center of the wake. Riding out, the same smile that settled onto her lips when she started, forms on her again. Full circle. It's done. The taste of salty air flooding her senses, the sweet taste of victory on her lips. The champ has emerged. She stepped into the encounter, fully faced the dangerous energy pounding through the ocean, took her position and proceeded through the chaotic surge storming around her, coming out the other side victorious. It did not take her under. The champ, still standing in the end. Standing in victory. The crowd standing in awe. Hearts moved and impacted, feeling the surreal moment of timelessness accompanying the witness of pure and clean athleticism.

CHAPTER THREE

HOW TRAINING EFFECTS THE BODY

T raining with intelligence, truly, is honoring the inherent intelligence housed in our body's internal mechanism, harnessing its release toward the target of peak performance. It is learning to work in cooperation with our design, allowing a congruence to flow from the inside out. A finely tuned athlete resonates.

Resonance. What does it mean to resonate? It is an athlete aligning deeply with their sport. It is two separate pieces to an interaction brought together, creating incredible harmony. For the athlete, it's what we see when their skill matches the demand of the sport. Integrating, coming together in a manner that builds one on another, an athlete and their sport showcase the champ within like no other.

Resonance, the harmony within our body, flows out in the sport we play. Resonance is internal, bringing together the many components within us that are involved in athletic work. Like a harmonious connection singing different musical notes but in beautiful harmony, the systems and functions involved in athletic work come together in an orchestral expression that spectators enjoy from the stadium seats. Internal resonance is developed in the crucible of training. The body practicing and learning, relearning and fine-tuning, with each training session. Developing systems integration. Resonating. Becoming more efficient, the athlete building from within. The flow of internal work becoming smooth, precise, clean, uncomplicated. Resonance and efficiency working hand in hand. The preparation in training is the process of building an athlete from the inside out.

Resonance is external, bringing what is within the athlete out and into harmony with their sport. The sport, being the showcase and backdrop of an athlete's internal development, creating an action and reaction relationship. The finely tuned athlete, matching his or her capabilities and movements with the demands of their sport. The sport, challenging the capabilities of the athlete in the show of the game. Creating resonance, in peak performance training, causes a oneness between the athlete and their sport. Internal systems primed, singing in harmony, the finely tuned athlete comes alive with passion and life at the start of their game. Eager to engage. It's more than a task. It's a oneness, a sense of deep unity. Complete resonance from the inside out. Complete resonance from within the athlete to its outer limits within the game. The impact of what is inside extending out, preparing for the impact and response of sport engagement.

IMPACT - THE DEFINING RELATIONSHIP BETWEEN SPORT AND ATHLETE

The power of relationship. How does it play out in sport? The energy flow from the athlete and the energy response from the sport culminate in a continuum of energy transfer. Force produced and received. Impact. For the athlete, this is an ebb and flow between extending and receiving impact as the sport is played out.

Impact is the power of an athlete's presence in the game of sport. It is the force production of the body being released into the game. Energy is released and then received in an athlete through sport engagement. With energy release in a game, force is produced and exerted on a sporting medium and then rebounded back to the athlete. This is the interaction of sport.

Sport is the interaction of energy. Energy bounding between one participant and another, one athlete and their sporting surface. While in some sports, we have opponents and opposing teams, in other sports, we have an athlete showcasing their athletic presence on a sporting surface. Think of running, surfing, skiing and snowboarding. The energy rebound, in these sports, is solely in the surface and equipment used to express athletic skill. While the impact may look different in different sports, there is a similar thread coursing through every sport. It is the thread of impact, the thread of energy transfer. It is this energy transfer that creates the relationship between a sport and the athlete.

THE INTERNAL RESONANCE OF SYSTEMS INTEGRATION

Peak performance is predicated on systems integration. Integration is the smooth cooperation of the many parts involved in peak performance. How do the systems that function in our athletic work integrate? Internally, there are two sides to our athletic work: the action and the reaction. It is the energy expenditure and the energy received. It is the power to impact and be impacted. Integration of our athletic work coincides with the two sides expressed in our sporting relationship. The athlete extends and receives, acting and sensing, impacting and being impacted. That integration, the smooth cooperation, is led and tied together by our nervous system. The autonomic nervous system turns on the athletic drive that creates our impact in the game. The central and peripheral nervous system produce and receive impact during the game.

The internal resonance of an athlete begins in the nervous system. Its electrical current organizing and directing systems and functions, varied and wide in the body, bringing them under the same purpose and goal. Smooth systems integration. Cooperating well. Flowing with ease. Extending further than the electrical connection, systems integration requires each part of the system to not only work together but also do their part well. The art of systems integration is the resonance of each cell, each organ, each system involved. From the depth, from the minute, from the microscopic to the grand display of athletic excellence, the crowd erupting, gasping in awe as the champ moves beyond the finish line.

Systems integration is the foundation of an athlete's skill set. Comprehensive and complete training sets an athlete up for the greatest success. To spend time overtly focused on one system involved in athleticism and forget the others is similar to developing the point guard at the neglect of the other team roles on a basketball team. What good is a point guard alone? Conversely, what good is muscle strength alone? It is powerless without integration with the other systems. It is powerless without the smooth cooperation of the nervous system. It is powerless without the brain. Athleticism is more than strength, flexibility and power. It is full body systems integration. It is worth repeating: ***Peak performance is predicated on systems integration.***

Integration in the human body is like exponential increase in mathematical calculations. Truly, the whole of the parts is exponentially greater and more powerful than the parts alone. As we discuss and develop understanding of the parts, keep in mind that the finished product, systems integration, is an efficient coordination of these parts and this is what we see as we witness the pristine and clean athleticism of a well-trained athlete. While integration creates smooth operation in the body, efficiency focuses and harnesses the energy in system operations. Both efficiency and integration are needed for the athlete to truly resonate in their sport.

THE DEVELOPMENT OF ATHLETIC EFFICIENCY

Harnessing peak performance is about creating clean energy exchange in the game of sport. Efficiency in an athlete is the focused expression of energy. The chaotic and undisciplined energy release is akin to working hard, and yet, missing the mark. It is the runner expending more energy in unnecessary movements, extra bounce, exaggerated toe off and vertical lift during the running continuum. Building efficiency in an athlete is moving them from choppy, hard and overwhelming in the face of challenge to an athletic expression of smooth, ease and overcoming. With competence and confidence built in the crucible of training, efficiency is built as the inherent intelligence develops over time. It is the body's nature to develop. The inherent intelligence does its perfect and maturing work with progressive challenge. As peak performance training does the work of building internal resonance, expressing energy, retrieving energy and cleaning obstacles to the energy exchange of sport takes place. Clean expression. Finely tuned. Resonated. Integrated. Efficient.

INTEGRATION AND EFFICIENCY - BUILDING RESONANCE FROM THE INSIDE OUT

Combining integration with efficient energy use, athletic expression becomes unified. The resonance reverberating from every cell involved. A well known Olympic skater comes to mind. Her performance is a distinct example of integration and efficiency. Nancy Kerrigan. Her blade pressing onto the ice, gliding forward. A beautiful picture of resonance, as one blade presses forward and then the other, igniting speed, body gracefully gliding along the ice. Turning, her feet move synchronously and then separately as the progression of her triple triple combination is prepared. The centripetal force whirling her as her feet lift in the powerful force of her legs. Power and grace. Body relaxed, flowing and yet, controlled and powerful. Landing, her blade skates the surface while the other foot whips behind her, lifting her again. Centripetal force reverberating. Resonance releasing. One more graceful lift and she glides out with ease and composure as her feet land yet again. The power of a resonant and efficient athlete played out before our eyes in the game of sport.

How does one develop athletic resonance? The ease with which an athlete moves within any given sport is developed in the crucible of training. Intelligent training. Intelligent training creates resonance by being resonant itself. It is both integrated and efficient, progressive and intelligent, working with the design of the body, working with the design of the sport, blending those two into excellence of movement. Resonant.

INTELLIGENT TRAINING

Training is both progressive and intelligent. Progressive and intelligent work steadily elevates an athlete's abilities over time. While it is intelligent in its ability to match and challenge the physiology in an athlete, it is progressive in its steady increase in the training challenge according to the athlete's improving abilities. Designed to "up the anty" over and over, to progressively build an athlete's resistance to challenge so much so that continued athletic growth requires progressively greater challenge, the key to effective training is to create a constructive training effect. It is to meet the athlete at the current level of ability and apply a training stimulus, stretching beyond that level, allowing the athlete to grow and empower into the next level.

ADAPTATION IS THE TRAINING EFFECT

Our body is designed to overcome and adapt. It is designed to overcome challenge, stress and difficulty. The goal of training is to create an intelligent and progressive demand on the body that will strengthen its ability to meet the challenge of sport. This is the principle of adaptation at work. Adaptation is the training effect. As the body responds to the demand, challenge and stress of training, adaptation is taking effect.

Challenges build the champ within. When faced with the desire to resign or retreat, remember that every challenge intelligently faced is the fire that cleans the inner obstacles of the champ within you. Surrounding yourself with the supports that move you toward the finish line, that encourage the emerging development of your inner champ, is wise. While there is encouragement internally from the deep love of sport, every athlete gets weary. To reach the summit of peak potential, a tribe of real and abiding support is helpful. The voices of those closest to you, believing in you, cheering you, investing in your development, encouraging you when the journey gets difficult is what helps keep an athlete engaged in the crucible of training.

Adaptation is the internal intelligence within the body, responding to the challenge. It is the physiology and systems, developing and improving. Do you know that, when the body is healthy, it naturally does this? Let it intelligently work for you, creating powerful adaptations, as you intelligently create the training effect.

Intelligent training leads to the activation of the quiet mechanisms of the intelligence within you. When training is applied in such a manner as to harness this quiet intelligence in an athlete, the training and the athlete resonate and build a steady foundation of athleticism.

Resonating in training leaves no training effort and its effect a waste of energy or time. The love of sport. The love of challenging your body. A lifetime of progressive challenge becomes enjoyable in the power of resonant training because resonant training limits burnout. Like a newborn child reaching for their next level in curious enjoyment, every level of our athletic adventure is marked with deep and curious joy when viewed in the long range lens of deep respect and love for movement, adaptation and the freedom to express that in sport. Steering the training effect into resonant adaptation secures the growth and steady progression of athletic abilities.

THE POWER OF ADAPTATION - STEERING THE TRAINING EFFECT

In discussing resonant adaptation, a word of caution about the steering power of adaptation is important. The tough reality is that adaptation works in both directions, working either for us or even against us if we are not careful. While it can be powerfully resonant, causing us to reach further, soar higher and stand on summits beyond our previous abilities, adaptation can also become dissonant. Dissonant adaptation creates a breakdown in systems integration and efficiency. A negative training effect takes place and the effort expended works against our desires and goals. Dissonant adaptation occurs among healthy individuals in two ways: via under training or overtraining. Finding the sweet spot of training keeps its effect resonating and working for the athlete.

Creating a resonant and intelligent challenge builds a response designed to overcome that stress. With under-training, there is a consistent retreat from a challenge that lowers the body's ability to engage and overcome it. Without challenge, we become weak. Instead of producing peak performance, the opposite, the loss of potential, takes effect. A defeated champ, a resigned champ, a champ that sadly gave up and let go is the result of that retreat. This is the dissonance of under training and demotivation. Discouragement. The breakdown in the emotion brain, tanking potential in self destructive fear and anxieties. The resignation of potential.

The other side of dissonant training is overtraining. Driven into perfectionism and fearful striving, pushing the body well beyond its challenging limits in an effort to shortchange the process leads to burnout and break down. The mindset of overtraining is moving beyond constructive and progressive gain and into a cheating gain. While there is nothing wrong with developing, growing and gaining athletic skill, the motive to build that skill plays out in our process of development. When the motive is to pridefully stand over another, the emotion brain slips into the destructive zone and begins motivating and moving our actions into the distraction of destructive competitiveness. Seeking the breakdown of another to build one's own sense of status and accomplishment leads the athlete away from what they have control over; themselves and their training regimen. The result of all that distracted and misplaced energy expenditure is personal breakdown. Destruction. From the inside out, destructive motives lead to breakdown and burnout. Injuries. Lack of training focus. Extraneous energy expenditure.

The reason why we train is just as valuable as the training itself. Guarding the motive, the love of sport and the love of athletic development keeps the mind centered and focused on what an athlete has control over; themselves and their training regimen. There is only one way to build the champ within. The athlete's power to change is centered on their performance. Did you ever notice a powerful athlete in the lead during a sporting event? Do you ever see them looking at anyone? What is their focus? Think about it. Have you seen what happens to a second place competitor at times? Do you see them staring at the rival in front of them? They've lost focus. Energy expended that does not necessarily serve their best performance undermines their ability. Motives matter. Focus matters.

CHOOSING POSITIVE ADAPTATION & RESONANCE

While adaptation is alarming and has the power to create a negative training effect, in reality, it is also deeply encouraging. It means we can exercise a choice in the direction we'd like to go. We have the power to choose our path. It is encouraging because our bodies are designed to overcome stress as we engage with the challenges of training. If we are willing to show up and let the body do its intelligent work, adaptation will work for us.

Applying the stress of intelligent training strengthens us to meet the demand of our sport. If we understand this about our body, we will be better equipped to work with their processes, allowing the inherent work to work for us, not against us. We can either flow in the currents of the ocean or flow against them. Much the same with training. We can work really hard against the natural and intelligent design within us or we can work smart and flow with it. Let's train intelligently. Let's stir the champ within.

Our body, much like a silent warrior, lying dormant. The lion roar of which is our inherent and original capabilities, our potential untapped, waiting for the challenge. It is the dormant champ, deciding whether to rise or resign when the challenge comes. Deciding whether to meet it head on, step into the game and make an impact or to remain untapped, unchallenged, reducing itself with every retreating step. To rise or resign. Everyone comes to a fork in the road. Everyone has a choice.

Waking that lion, stirring the heart of that inner warrior, is the purpose of intelligent training. Why not let the warrior rise? Why not release the sound of the roar within you? Why not ignite the fire of a fully alive way of life, crashing into our world with a powerful and incredible impact like none other, re-verberating for decades after you are gone? Why not let the rip-ple effect of your existence leave an athletic legacy in your wake for years to come? Why not? Why would you not? Is that de-sire stirring in you yet? I hope so. Shake off that dust. You were meant to rise.

THE TRIAD SWEET SPOT

The sweet spot of training is producing a constructive training effect, powerfully steering the athlete into positive adaptation and progressive skill development. Healthy, reso-nant training is constructive, it is foundational and it builds lay-er upon layer in skill set. Destructive and dissonant training is unhealthy and unproductive, often undermining an athlete's de-velopment. In a dissonant or negative training effect, the energy expended is not harnessed for peak performance, but is out of control. It flows in any direction without guidance or purpose. An athlete in peak performance requires energy focus. Keeping an athlete in the center of the sweet spot in training maintains that focus, allowing the work done to serve the purpose of the training rather than undermine and sabotage it.

Specifically, the triad of that sweet spot is threefold. It is the sport, the athlete and the relationship between the two. It is a triad in the three following ways: 1) in harnessing the inherent intelligence within the inner workings of the athlete's body, 2) in intelligently assessing the sporting demands within an athlete's specific sport of choice, and 3) in intelligently matching the athlete and the sport to build a oneness, a resonance between the two. Building resonance between an individual athlete and their sport requires understanding of both to blend them well. One component in this equation, the athlete, has characteristics that are generalizable according to research. Yet, there are also characteristics that are highly individual, thus, there is an art to developing athletic skill as well as a science!

THE SCIENCE AND ART OF TRAINING

Similar to physical rehab, peak performance training is both an art and a science. An art because the context one applies the science into, that of a diverse human being, is like a fingerprint and not exact in the way science esteems to achieve. Science is distinct, objective, standardized and measurable. Humans are not all on the same continuum, they are not robotic machines manufactured in the exact same manner. To apply a science into the context of mysterious and complete diversity requires an artistic ability. We must remember that science is designed to impact a living, breathing, organic and developing human, often with a history and unique genetic make-up that has implications for each decade of training. The art of application lends respect to this unique variable.

Peak Performance Training not only considers the science but also the art in its application. The science is what we are able to measure and become concrete on its effect. It impacts the art of humanity, which is not able to be completely quantified, definitively standardized or concretely measured. There are aspects of our humanity that are, but the totality of our humanity is not. This, the totality of our humanity, is the artistic canvas that our science impacts. With that said, appreciating the intelligent design of the athlete's body while maintaining a healthy respect for its inability to be perfectly duplicated and copied adds flexibility to the training strategies. Studying the individual athlete is an aspect of the sweet spot triad of training that helps close the gap in what is known about the human body and what is specific to the individual athlete.

EFFECTIVE TRAINING - DRIVING THE TRAINING EFFECT

Effective training requires a constructive challenge and an adequate recovery to assimilate the internal body changes needed to adapt to the challenge! What does this mean? Effective training requires correct assessment of an athlete's abilities, a training challenge that stretches that ability and a recovery that allows for that stretch to build real substance in the athlete's body. To layer it even more, effective training requires a focus of both the training challenge and training recovery that serves athletic vision. There are two parts interacting; the athlete and the sporting context. Both assessments are connected by and become integrated through training. One assessment details an athlete's current abilities, the other assessment details the sporting context. The training brings the relationship between the two into peak performance.

When there is a mismatch between the training, the athlete and the sporting context, training becomes less effective. Less intelligent. What makes it intelligent is the match. Remember, that an athlete engaging with their sport is about a relationship. It is them bringing the energy and force of their existence into the game. Developing a training regimen that builds peak performance is respecting this relationship and building a resonant impact within it. In a nutshell, it is catching the sweet spot between each of them. It is aiming the training sweet spot for the athlete into the sporting context. It is designing the training regimen based on the analysis of the sport. And it is staying in that sweet spot as the athlete progresses.

THE SWEET SPOT OF THE TRAINING CHALLENGE

The sweet spot for an athlete's training remains in the bounds of constructive growth and aimed within the context of sport. In avoiding the slip into under-training or over-training, the athlete progressively builds a solid and more complete foundation. This foundation is built by both the external parameters of the training and the internal parameters of the body's response to the training. Relating the training to the body and the body's response to the training helps define the boundaries of the training regimen. As the athlete becomes more conditioned, these boundaries shift with them. The internal parameter is the conditioning zone of an athlete's body. It is the boundaries and limits of ability within the athlete themselves. It is the body's ability to handle stress and remain in a constructive, building response. Pressing beyond those boundaries places the athlete into the destructive zone and out of the sweet spot of training. Remember, the sweet spot is designed to keep the athlete from sabotaging their own efforts. Every expenditure of energy is being used to build and not undermine by overstepping.

Conversely, the external parameter, the stressor, is the training stimulus. The training challenge. It serves to progressively challenge the body's limit, pressing just beyond it to reach for the next level in training. In rehab language, we call this fine line the "therapeutic zone". In training language, I'd call this the "peak training zone".

Recall that the body's response to the challenge of training is adaptation. The body's adaptations are not only muscular but occur in every system that is engaged with the physical exertion and effort. As the body is impacted by the challenge, it takes it in and processes it on a deep level within us. It is like it does a wide scale assessment during and after the exercise training stimulus and begins making adjustments and fine-tuning systems, building more substances associated with creating an overcoming response and preparing itself for the next time it is confronted with this level of challenge. If this doesn't make you stand in a state of awe or get your head spinning about the intelligence inherent in your body, let's stop right here. Take your finger and place it on the inside of your wrist.

Do you feel a pulse? Are you alive? How can this realization not hit you square in the head with a new level of respect for your body?! It is truly phenomenal!

Adaptation, like mentioned earlier, has a caution to it. It can work for us or against us. For instance, in a disease state, adaptation weakens and de-conditions the body and rehab is required to shift the direction of adaptation and recover our baseline condition. In a peak state, adaptation strengthens and conditions the body to press the limits of our current capabilities into excellent expressions of physical ability. The difference is in the direction of the adaptation. This is a broad definition with a large effect, toggling between elite and peak performance and progressive and chronic illness. In training, more specifically, adaptation regressions can effect training during and even between seasons on a lesser scale. To keep adaptation working for us and not against us while we are in a training season, there is a delicate balance between training stimulus and recovery. Too much recovery, and the scales shift negatively in adaptation. Too little recovery, and well, then we have overtraining and that is another area to avoid altogether.

CONNECTING THE ATHLETE TO THE SPORT

Effective training includes two assessments and a leadership focus. The first assessment is that of the athlete. A full medical evaluation is advisable to clear of any injuries. Then, an athletic assessment inclusive of all body systems is prudent.

Next, an assessment of the sport and its physics dynamics, which body systems need to be engaged and trained and how the athlete is able to develop within that sporting context. Leadership through coaching or training requires a vision for training. Once the detailed assessments of both the athlete and the sport are completed, there then becomes the athlete's goals, the reality of the athlete's abilities and the natural talent within the athlete. Is this sport a good match for this athlete? Is it the best match? Do they enjoy the sport? Does their body have a lean toward the demands of the sport? Will this sport set up this athlete for success or failure based on their athletic profiling and predisposition? Does the athlete want to participate because they enjoy it and don't care about a perfect match? What is important to the athlete? Does the athlete want to find a match in a sport that fits them more or do they love the sport and really aren't concerned about it? This is the part of the assessment that is highly personal to the athlete. Leadership takes this information and develops a plan with realistic goals and expectations. Leadership is honest about an athlete's abilities and inherent predisposition without being absolute or dogmatic about the outcome. There are always anomalies!

Leadership connects the athlete to the sport. This connection is done after the evaluation of both. It is the planning stage. It is the place of taking the components and ordering them into a training regimen. The training regimen is the avenue that an athlete begins to become efficient and resonant in their sporting relationship. It is the delicate dance between stretch and rest. Stimulus and recovery. Challenge and chill.

THE SWEET SPOT OF THE TRAINING RECOVERY

So, what's the deal with recovery? Well, recovery is the time our body goes into fierce adaptation mode. It is building, manufacturing, developing and harnessing your body's systems to perform stronger at the next challenge. It is literally where your body builds peak performance. Disrespecting this is like saying, "I just want to stay mediocre even though I am working my tail off!" Who says that?! No one. It's ludicrous. What is important is to look at recovery with a healthy attitude. Recover like a Champ! Refrain from undermining your body's preparation for your next challenge. Let it develop and then engage again at another training stimulus until the body adapts at that level. Then, engage again at another level of stimulus until the process of adaptation has had its perfect work there as well. Guess what? This is the process of developing *foundational athleticism*. From the beginning to the culmination. Birthing, emerging, becoming, developing, rising. A legend. A legacy. Coming full circle. The victory lap of a champion's life is more than the accolades. It's a life well-lived.

THE EMERGING OF A CHAMP

THE BIRTHING OF A CHAMPION

Deep within the heart (emotion brain), lies a dormant champion. Here he is. Young, impressionable. Clinging to his surfboard. Unsure who to trust, his mind is caught in the sea of impounding wave upon wave, as one thought interrupts another. Whirling with doubt and fear, thoughts scrambling for decisive action, for direction, for guidance. Slowly standing under the pressure, abruptly turning his head to swing his hair from his face, shaking the sand from his legs. Determined, he looks out at the ocean. Studying its rhythms, imagining riding through its tunneling force. Looking down at his board, his connecting source to the ocean, appreciation and deep regard flooding through him as he thinks of his connection to this aspect of the earth. It is a passion he is unable to articulate. All he knows is that, when he is on his board, in sync with its surface, everything feels right. Feels like home.

Standing still, battling his doubts and fears, his decision is firm. "This is what my life's work will be", he whispers to himself. The ocean calling him in ways he doesn't dare share aloud for it all seems so uncanny, so unreal. What is this force pulling me toward it? An undeniable attraction, a draw that grows stronger and stronger, overpowering his apprehensions. The doubts fade. A deep resignation, a giving over to the call and beckoning of the ocean. The wind picking up around him, steady in the coming storm. It's coming. Looking up, he sees the storm clouds forming. Quietly, he bows his head. This is more than the storm. This is the beginning of a prevailing force in the face of the storm.

THE CHAMP REVEALED

Against the backlash of dark clouds, his life's work riding the wave of victory in a culmination of transformation. The storm, driving the energy of his sport, now released and birthing new developments, new technology. The victorious champion. The trophies, the accolades, the awards are sweet reminders to something so deep. Words cannot begin to express its depth. But he knows. In that inner place of deep thought, the depth of his soul, fully satisfied in the fulfillment of a lifelong commitment.

Thinking back to that young moment on the sand, recalling the trepidation in his heart, smiling at the sustaining power of the call. Full circle. It's coming full circle. The emerging champ at that first moment, stuck in a decision. Looking back, he wonders if he actually made that decision or if it made the decision, moving his heart. The mechanisms of the movement in the ocean seemed to somehow reach out and move him, birthing a lifelong connection to its honor, wellbeing and sanctity. His love runs deep as the ocean depth, fighting for her, advocating for her, standing for her. Perhaps that is why she chose him. As much as he needed her, she also needed him. While making her his friend, she exalted him to the high places of honor. Wisdom inherent in the ocean's depth, inherent in the earth's rhythms calling out to him. Deep unto deep.

Unbeknownst to him, his journey was so much deeper than he first realized. She took him to the depths, soared him on her heights and released him into the wildest, torrential forces surrounding him. Released and riding out in a blaze of glory in a myriad of ways. Surfboards collected, memories cemented, the ocean brought life to his life. It developed him as he developed our view and respect of her. Standing in the sand, years later, looking out over the horizon. The force of his impact, his athletic presence, going beyond the wave. Deep peace settling in, he steps in. It never gets old.

THE ATHLETIC LEGACY

When we meet athletes that have been training for 3 years, 5 years, 10 years and they have built a steady foundation of healthy growth and development, we will stand in awe of their ability to do very difficult things with seemingly little effort. ***This is the power of progressive training.***

Progressive training is the mindset of long term thinking and vision within athleticism. It is the beginning of an athlete's legacy and lifetime pursuit of excellence in physical expression and in their sport, depending on how specific the athlete has chosen to be. Progressive training requires periodic assessments that include understanding of an athlete's development in their body. It is the difference between a 13 year old, a 22 year old, 35 year old, 49 year old, 75 year old and 90 year old athlete. There are different considerations to acknowledge at each decade of life. There is a deep understanding of the growth and development process that takes a body into full maturity as well as the aging process that begins to affect our system's over time. Peak performance is really about matching an athlete's body and all its considerations with the sport demands. Those considerations are as complex as the body itself! The athlete's body is a changing agent over time which include factors such as athletic goals, medical history, injury history, training history, stage of development and current training abilities.

The ability to establish a foundation of training earlier in an athlete's life, the better. When we are in our first decade, there are some powerful opportunities to create habits that set a foundation for life. It's like painting on a clean canvas. There is so much impression and simple receptivity to the new activities. The learning is quicker and the activities become automatic. The downside to this, of course, is that if we have been trained in a way that is not constructive to athletic development, later on in life, we will need to spend time unlearning those faulty training inputs to learn again a new way. Prevention is better than recovery. Although, thank goodness for recovery because where would any of us really be without it? No one has a perfect foundation built. *One of the goals of Train with Intelligence is to bring this awareness to the forefront and train our young athletes on a foundation that will serve*

them for life. It is also to take athletes further along in the process through an untraining/retraining stimulus to help them recover their peak potential!

Each decade of life presents a new way to approach training. And, of course, this is affected by how well a person was conditioned prior to reaching that decade of life. A highly conditioned individual from their youth will be much younger in their body processes than someone who has not trained until their third or fourth decade. Needless to say, training at any decade will begin to produce amazing results and is worth jumping in at any time.

THE SPARK OF ATHLETIC LEGACY

How did the birth of a champion happen in this scenario? How did the call, the moment of decision, translate into fulfillment? Take a look at what happened in him as he wrestled with the doubt and fear. It was the spark of a sporting relationship, coupled with the realization that wisdom, insight and training was needed to secure the fulfillment of that vision hitting his heart. He may not have realized it then. But, vision happened. An organic birthing, a spark of a new beginning, a lifelong pursuit and journey that would lead his steps like someone driven by vision. A true entrepreneur. He caught the vision before he understood the mechanisms behind his fingerprinted and unique make up. It also caught him in an encountered moment between what was in him and what he was looking at. The relationship sparking between an athlete and his sport. The fears, the doubts settling into him with a realization that mentorship was in his future. The settled resignation. The acceptance.

Driven by vision. He caught the vision. The vision caught him. It was a match made, quite possibly beyond understanding, quietly entering his world and gently blowing its breeze through that salty hair of his. Did he know? Perhaps he knew something was extraordinary. Yet, one day, his eyes would open and the realization of a bigger vision and purpose would become clear in his vision. The power of the ocean turning his attention, steering him toward a legacy and destiny that he would one day discover at the culmination of it all. The adventurous journey into the heart of a champ, from the birth to the culmination. Built within. The champ ignited and fully alive. Depth and meaning deepening year after year. The champ isn't a trophy. It's what is built within extending out in reverberating and resounding impact. In a blaze of glory, the champ revealed. What was buried deep within was brought to the surface for all to see.

TRAINING CONSIDERATIONS

The connecting cord between an athlete another sporting relationship is their training regimen. Looking at the board, we see one of the main aspects of his training. To intelligently train, one must study the board. It is the device used to connect the athlete to the wave. In training, looking at the device mechanics is crucial. How does the device connect into the sport, how does it interact with the athlete, what is the purpose of the device? An in depth look at the device helps understand the method that the athlete engages the sport.

To effectively connect the athlete into the sport, each piece of the sport must be considered. This includes the athlete in all his or her unique design and abilities, the devices in the sport and all the aerodynamics and physics involved in its use, and finally the surface of the sport. In this case, these three are Kelly Slater and his training history, medical history and current abilities, his board and the purpose of its design, and the physics of the wave. Once these pieces are thoroughly considered on their own, the next step is to connect and integrate the pieces. Systems integration is not only within an athlete's body, it is played out in the effect of that body in their sporting context. The training regimen must include all three considerations in development individually and in smooth development collectively. Leaving any one of these pieces of analyses amiss and there will be holes in the foundation of the training. There are opportunities missed, peak abilities unrealized and potential untapped.

While the training analysis occurs in a champion surfing example here, it is the same context of consideration for all sports. Intelligent training considers the context and develops a comprehensive understanding of the sport prior to developing its peak performance training plan. The phrase "let's not put the cart before the horse" comes to mind. Setting an athlete up for success is a step by step process with an order that prioritizes a deep understanding of the sport, the individual athlete, and the relationship between them.

TRAINING IS BOTH CHALLENGE & RECOVERY

Peak performance training includes both the training challenge and recovery. It is an interplay between both. Training stimulus is the active work of training. It is where the sweat, physical challenges and pressing of our current capabilities occur. Training recovery is the passive work of training. Passive is a term that I have grappled with in this definition as it does not adequately grab what is happening internally in the body. Internally, our bodies are extremely active, but the biological processes that occur in recovery require us to actively rest from our training stimulus, hence the term "passive". Without recovery, the stimulus, or the challenge, is not able to complete its perfect work in our bodies. The perfect work of adaptation.

There is a delicate balance between both training stimulus and training recovery. When these are not attuned, dissonance occurs in the body much like the sound of clashing cymbals and disorganized instrumentation in an orchestra. We know that sound can be made, but when it's not attuned, it becomes more destructive than helpful or even enjoyable. On another note, dissonance in the body creates a lack of "ease", or what healthcare professionals would call "disease". Disease states occur in our body when the opposite occurs with peak performance. It is the result of adaptation gone awry and away from the direction of Peak Performance.

Peak Performance is attuning these two aspects of training to create an integrated training effect. An integrated training effect reduces injuries, increases morale and motivation, helps athletes truly enjoy the physical expression of their abilities, and sets a foundation for lifelong training and momentum. So, what happens when these two pieces are not attuned? Or, put another way, what happens when they don't function in a way that supports and builds on one another?

Well, when there is too much training stimulus and too little training recovery, the training becomes destructive, creating harm, injury and potential burnout in the body. When a training stimulus is not adequate enough to challenge the body and the training recovery is too long, the result is de-conditioning and a reduced ability to reach full potential. Peak performance training lies in the center of these two extremes and represents a tension between training activity and training recovery. For each athlete, this tension is very individual. It is dependent on many factors, including their level of training, their body's ability to recover, nutritional factors, among other factors.

"Peak performance training lies in the center of these two extremes and represents a tension between training activity and training recovery."

STIMULUS & RECOVERY DEFINED FURTHER

The training program includes both the stimulus and the recovery. Stimulus is the training event, while recovery is the body's response to that event. It's the training effect. The event and its response. Cause and effect in operation. Stimulus is the demand and call to action on the body. Recovery is the body's refueling and adaption to that demand.

What are the various types of training stimuli? Strength training. Flexibility training. Balance training. Metabolic training. Endurance training. Core strength training. Sport specific training. There's a training event for every mobility piece of our body's function.

How is a training program designed? We've discussed already the triad sweet spot of training. Assessment of an athlete includes assessing the athlete, the sport and the athlete-sport interaction. A training program is designed by integrating these three assessments and then reassessing them periodically. The reassessment is designed to keep the athlete moving toward the goal and context of their sport. With that in mind, let's discuss each type of training individually. Much of the athlete assessment will include areas of needed improvements in the contexts of these types of training. An athlete that doesn't need real time reactionary balance in their sport may score low and weak on that type of balance assessment, but it ranks as low priority in the context of their training regimen because of its low demand in the sport chosen. A training program needs to drive its assessments into the priorities of the sporting context. This is the triad sweet spot of training. It is the integration of the athlete's abilities, training assessments and sporting demands. It is creating a oneness between the athlete and the demands of the sports. Resonance.

TRAINING SEASONS

As the foundations of an athlete are built, there is an ebb and flow between cross training and specific sports training. The cross training seasons are where the general foundations of athleticism are built within an athlete. Weaknesses are honed in on metabolically, nutritionally, and in any other neuromuscular and musculoskeletal manner. If there are gaps, they are filled in this season. The foundation training focus is width. Well rounded athletes build wide as well as deep in their abilities. Progressive seasons of training take the foundation wider and deeper over time until the foundation is so strong, it can withstand great force and stress without flinching.

While cross training builds wide, sport specific training builds deep. Focusing intently on the specific sporting demands, the training is pruned to fine-tune and build sport specific resonance. Standing on the foundation of wide and deep athletic ability, the athlete is then able to launch to greater heights of achievement and ability. Laying the foundation in seasons of training reduces injuries, builds resilience, enhances motor memory and builds movement precision. Like a sharpening tool, progressive training, in and out of certain seasons, continues to sharpen the athlete into a fine point of focused impact for their game of sport.

CROSS TRAINING

Two types of training seasons involved in the training program design for athletes are the cross-training and sport specific training seasons. While periodization is the organization of training seasons within a year, the type of training within the periodization takes an athlete through an ebb and flow of physical development. It not only gives the athlete's body a rest from the fine motor demands in sport specific training, it builds a wide base of stability in cross training seasons. The organization of training seasons is inclusive of pre-season training, season training, post-season training and cross-training. Of course, these seasons can be altered especially if there is not a specific athletic sport one is working toward in the beginning of their athletic career and endeavor.

In preparing an athlete for sport, especially in younger years, it is wise to work at setting a foundation of motor learning, and developing a wide base of ability to reduce injury and build resilience in a body. In the beginning of athletic pursuit, it is important to spend more time in cross training to build a solid foundation prior to launching into specific training. Remember, it is the core of stability that provides the base for specificity. If the stable base is not built adequately, the specific and fine motor skills required for the details of sport fall apart.

What is cross training? It is seasons of training that are more general and not as sport specific as other seasons. They include training that focuses on building cardiovascular, lung and peripheral efficiency as well as strength, power and stamina in the manner their sports requires but with a variable mode of training. So, if your sport is surfing, you'll need some anaerobic and aerobic training because the upper body work of paddling out against the current is intense work, yet the length of time between sets and intense activity is prolonged in a heat. In surfing, you'll also need a lot of neuromuscular training that targets the pathways that engage during the sport itself. When you are in a specific training season, the focus and goal is on very specific movement patterns. When you are in a cross-training season, you'll still want to focus on the same systems but the difference is you'll train them across many modes of training.

General cross training seasons train the body within the same system engagement but across many modes of work. It is developing a foundation in training and allowing the body the freedom of movement to dispel training injuries and give an athlete a broad athletic base. The more well-rounded an athlete becomes, the more stable the specificity of movement is. When there are seasons of too much specific training and too little cross training, injuries occur. Sadly, once an injury is in an athlete's history, there's recovery, but when we are talking of developing peak performance with a demand on the athlete's body of taking it to its absolute limit, those injuries create an impact on that ability in an athlete. They may not affect the recreational athlete, but they will affect an athlete that is reaching for elite level abilities. Having a healthy respect for cross training seasons, intelligent training principles, the complexities of the human systems involved in the sport, the type of medium the sport provides for the body to act upon and the way both that medium and the athlete relate to produce peak performance are all keys to unlocking and harnessing full potential in an athlete and setting a foundation for a legacy of athleticism. Athleticism does not need to be a fast and furious ride, quickly ending with a broken body for the remainder of an athlete's life. It may be that way with some sports due to the aggressive nature of certain games and the potential risk of contact injuries that are not as controlled for as in other sports or training regimens. Those are risks every athlete takes as they engage in their specific sport. Yet, minimizing injury with the right kind of training stimulus and creating powerhouse performance to conquer the sport medium is the goal of training. Reaching Peak Performance is not slamming a body through a treatment regimen. It is adequately assessing the context, both the human body's unique parameters in the athlete and the sporting surface, and then taking the athlete into a training regimen that stresses their systems just above their current level and in the direction of their particular athletic goal.

SPORT SPECIFIC TRAINING

Specificity in training is a training season focused on developing precision in the specific movements of your sport. Precision and efficiency for specific, complex and often whole body movement patterns involved in sport requires a training season to focus on this development. That is what sport specific training is for. The movements and demands of the sport are analyzed, integrated into the training and the athlete becomes attuned to these movements patterns through repetition. That repetition being the avenue for motor control and motor memory. For a basketball player, specific training would be developing the skill of handling the basketball on the court. For a surfer, it would be fine-tuning the balance reactions on a board with spontaneous force injections from the environment that a wave provides. For a biker, it would be bike mechanics, breathing, core and movements that reduce fatiguability with prolonged biking. For a runner, it would be development of proper running mechanics, focusing on the foot interaction with the ground and how the forces of the ground translate up the rest of the body. It would also be the efficiency in breathing, core activation and the balance between maintaining a relaxed state while being extremely active to use energy in a focused, efficient manner.

Remember that energy needs to be focused and harnessed for peak performance. Within the context of sport, that energy begins its deep focus in seasons of sport specific training.

What this means is that after an athletic assessment and a sports analysis is completed, a plan to develop maximal efficiency for the athlete's body systems that are specifically required for engagement in that sport needs to be developed. Think of harnessing energy like the difference between a beginner trying to swim and a seasoned athlete swimmer. The movements of the seasoned athlete are smooth, appear effortless and produce clean and quick action. Whereas the new athlete swimmer tends to be inefficient in their energy production, use of their body to engage in the sport and in their ability to act on the environment of the sport, which in this case is the water. There is evidence of a lot of effort being put into the task and not very much steady, sport specific movement as of yet. That's ok. That is actually a part of being a beginner.

Through the process of motor learning, the body becomes more efficient as training does its work. Remember, training develops efficiency specific to what one is training for. And motor learning is a key component to specificity of training. There is a general type of motor learning that one develops in cross training seasons. But, it is in specific seasons of training that motor learning begins to lay down habits of movement that are very important to sports. Think of it like learning to ride a bike. In the beginning, one has to think a lot about the tasks but very quickly, one is able to hold a discussion, wave at neighbors as they ride by, and ride a bike without really thinking about it all. This is motor learning. It is becoming so efficient in a complex motor task as to not think deliberately about it when doing so.

There is an amazing opportunity with specific training. If an athlete gets proper training in the beginning with motor learning, there will be an automatic process of peak performance. Yet, if the training is not ideal and the athlete spends time learning inefficient ways to do the specific and complex movements of their sport, it will be much more challenging to unlearn the habits of that training and re-establish new habits. And, even worse, if those habits of movement patterns have been repetitively acted out for a longer period of time, the deeper our brains lay down neural pathways. The deeper they are, the more challenging it will be to unlearn them. It can be done. But, it will add a training burden that would not be present when the training was done efficiently at the onset.

Specificity of training is taking complex movements in an athlete's sport and developing motor learning strategies until these movements become automatic without much thought. It's about developing precision. To do this, the training season needs to be focused on integrating the sporting demand with the athlete's body and systems. This includes complex movement patterns such as a baseball pitch or a soccer pass. It involves assessing the surface of the sport, the forces the body must move against, with or pass through as well as the aero-dynamics inherent in the equipment of the sport. Seasons of specific training match the athlete to the sport in as much detail as is possible.

FOUNDATIONAL TRAINING PROGRESSION

Training is done best by progressing through the same neuromuscular progressions that we progress through in our development. This is the general beginning of foundational training. Foundation training begins at the base of simple movements patterns and then progresses into more complex patterns. Training in a complex manner before building simpler movements sets an athlete up for injury. Developmentally, the human body first develops muscular control at the spine and core. Then, shoulder blades and hips and finally at the periphery, the arms and legs. Much the same in developing the strength of an athlete. Think about it all as being strong from the inside, at the core, to the outside, at the arms and legs.

There is an inherent intelligence in patterning the progression of foundational training after our normal developmental patterns. Our body develops like it does for a reason. Ankle strength was not developed before core control for a reason. Core control does not depend on ankle strength but the ankle does depend on certain stability at the core, does it not? What good is a strong ankle with a core that cannot hold itself aright? What good are the fine, more complex movements in the hand if the stabilizing strength of the core, shoulder and back are not there to support its expression and use? The complex, precision movements are developed on the foundation of stabilization. Stabilization begins at the center so that precision can express itself at the periphery. Foundational training patterned after this developmental sequence builds exponential strength and power in an athlete. The more solid the base, the more strength and force production is able to integrate through the system and discharge at the foot or hand, shoulder or hip, or whatever other body part the specific sport demands on an athlete. The point is, the more precision required, the greater the stability needed to express it well. Considering this training progression when building a training program builds deep as well as wide!

THE VISION FOR INTEGRATED ATHLETICISM

The power in integrated movement is muscles moving together and creating force together. It's similar to a team bringing the force of its compounded and integrated presence to the game versus a solo athlete game. A team working together brings more impact to the game. There is always more complication when integrating a team, but the dividends outweighs the investment. The same with the human body. When force production and it's fine-tuned execution is properly integrated in the body and all parts are working together well, there is a power that is profoundly greater than that of the parts. Training the body to move in integrated manner, engaging the base of its core and executing movement with the aide of more than one muscle primer helps an athlete maximize force production and power. It starts at the core, progresses through foundational training and produces clean and powerful movement that is greater than what is done with a lone muscle group.

ASYMMETRIC AND SYMMETRIC MOVEMENT PATTERNS

While some athletic events isolate muscle use more than most, such as in power lifting, most athletic sporting expressions are a wide combination of whole body strength and power movements. Think of the hockey player maintaining balance, skating across the ice, torquing the body to power drive the puck past the goalie. There's a lot of asymmetric coordination. It's not just stabilization of the body while isolating a single movement. While that is a feat in itself, we can appreciate the wide variety we see in athletic expression overall. Hence, why a well rounded training assessment is necessary to hit the mark of training for each athlete. Not only the assessment of the athlete in the game in general, but also the specific role of the athlete in any given game. This plays out even stronger with team sports, such as basketball or variety of events in track and field. On one team, the diversity of roles needs its own assessment and match to the specific athlete functioning in that role.

FOUNDATIONAL MOVEMENTS IN PROGRAM DESIGN

When designing any piece of an athlete's training program, it's important to remember the foundational basis of our movements. Core development first. Once this has a steady foundation, the next level is moving into taxing the core stability through limb dynamics. Simple, straight plane movements precede complex movement patterns. Tax the core by first maintaining limb dynamics in straight plane and simple movements until the skill set is safe and strong at its base. Then, complex movement patterns that move the limbs out of single muscle control planes is the next step.

Single muscle planes are the directions of movement with a predominant muscle action guiding the limb trajectory. Single joint planes are movements of a limb in which muscles work together for a common direction of movement. The most advanced movements are the complex movement patterns that do not have a predominant muscle activator or follow a single joint plane direction. Thus, they require a very high level of sophisticated coordination in muscles and joint movement. It would be quite unwise to begin training at that level of sophistication. Foundational training requires developing the most base skill, whether that is using that movement in strengthening, flexibility, balance, coordination, endurance or metabolic functioning.

COORDINATING TRAINING SEASONS

Seasons vary from athlete to athlete. Some athletes are all around, multi-sport athletes, some are intensely focused on one sport. Developing seasonal training will correspond well with the assessment of the athlete and their overarching year long sporting interactions. There is an ebb and flow to seasonal training. Being disciplined while strategic, and yet, creating room for creative play and expression is crucial for the athlete's overall health and wellness in sport. Crucial, not only for variety of movement and keeping injury low, but also for the mind, motivation and overall enjoyment of their sport. Athletes are meant to be both disciplined and creative, time-constrained and timeless. Allowing for a flow in and out of these expressions keeps an athlete in the game for life, securing the longevity and minimizing burnout.

Seasonal training is designed to create variety and the rhythms associated with that variety do best to take into account the way the brain operates. There are two sides to the brain. In athletics, especially in highly complex movement pattern sports, there is a very high demand placed on the brain. Seasons that vary and tap into the two types of brain functions keep the athlete balanced and fresh. One side of the brain is deeply engrossed in discipline, order, reason and logic. The other side is highly involved in timeless, creative expression. Seasons including this ebb and flow will feed the brain and empower it to ebb and flow within its sport.

TRAINING PROGRAM DEVELOPMENT

Developing a training program includes the triad analysis. The athlete, the sport dynamics and the relationship of the athlete to the sport. Once the training assessments are completed, the next step is to develop the training stimuli/challenge, training recovery plan, timeframe and season flow. The training assessments will help drive the areas of development in the seasons. Integrating the assessments is a leadership task. Remember that the training program is inclusive of both stimulus and recovery. Both are strategic to an athlete's development.

TRAINING STIMULI

When organizing a training stimulus program, there are many moving parts to include in this aspect of the program. Let's start with strength training.

Training is done best by progressing through the same neuromuscular progressions that we progress through in our development. It is foundational training. Foundation training begins at the base of simple movements patterns and then progresses into more complex patterns of strengthening. Training in a complex manner before building simpler movements sets an athlete up for injury.

Developmentally, the human body first develops muscular control at the spine and core. Then, shoulder blades and hips and finally at the periphery, the arms and legs. Much the same in developing the strength of an athlete. Think about it all as being strong from the inside, at the core, to the outside, at the arms and legs.

STRENGTH TRAINING

Muscles become strong by stressing them under forces of resistance. There are a myriad of ways our body is able to create force to accomplish this. Functional training, weight training, resistance band/tube training, to name a few.

STRENGTH TRAINING ALLEGORY - POWER

Hearing the sound of the start, toes pressing off and exploding powerfully out, the race is on. Arms pumping, legs pressing the body forward. One and then the other leading the trunk to the finish line. The chest pressing forward, the time called as the finish line is crossed. Over in seconds. Panting and gasping for breath. Walking, hands on hips, chest expanding, heart still racing. She looks back to check the times. Heart slowing, sweat pouring out as her body catches up and recovers. The champ has done it. Gold medal. 12.2 seconds. Bench-marked at the World Record. Elizabeth Robinson. 1928. The first female to run in the Olympic Track & Field games. Amsterdam. Historical. Legendary. Groundbreaking pioneer.

Two extremes of strengthening exist on the spectrum. On one end is this power and explosive expression of strength with maximum force developing in the muscles, yet only sustainable for a short time. This is powerful strength. On the other end of the strength spectrum is the type of strengthening that produces force in muscles over a longer period of time. This is enduring strength.

STRENGTH TRAINING ALLEGORY - ENDURANCE

Rounding through the relief station, halfway through her 55 mile race, taking her shoe off, her clubbed foot wrapped and bandaged. Smiling, she rehydrates and snacks while the volunteer re-bandages her foot, in awe of the paradox. The paradox of normal foot mechanics and endurance in the race. The paradox of a woman smiling, in pain, and unmoved in her pursuit of the remaining 22.5 miles. Her focus beyond the immediate, beyond the obvious discomfort, preparing for the next leg of her race. With determination, she rises, foot freshly bandaged and ready. Moving forward, placing one foot in front of the other in a steady stride, she begins her trek up the switch backs of the mountain for the next round. Brave. Enduring. Focused. She's off again, the volunteer watching as she presses up the trail and runs out of sight. Standing in awe, deep respect flooding the heart, the volunteer still. The excellence in the heart of an athlete revealed. A moment of silence and honor. Unnamed and unsung hero. The quiet force of her athletic presence persevering. Finishing her race.

Between the two extremes of power and endurance, there are a variety of athletic expressions. While our bodies are influenced by training, there is a genetic predisposition that influences our ability to flourish in certain types of training. Specifically, in the area of muscle strength, the DNA within us predisposes us to certain fiber types. Fiber types direct the type of predominant strength our muscles express, landing somewhere along the continuum of strength between the two extremes of explosive power and enduring power. Assessing an athlete takes these natural strengths into consideration when preparing a training program and operating within the sporting context.

FLEXIBILITY TRAINING

Muscles require strength to produce force. They also require extensibility to move freely and fully. Flexibility is the lengthening and agile aspect of a muscle. Creating athletic expression harnesses both muscle strength and muscle extensibility because movement is both free flowing and powerful. The athlete of strength and power is unrestricted when extensibility is conditioned. Muscles that move free of restrictions are free to express strength and power in the full range of mobility. A strong athlete without the ability to fully move is an athlete whose function in sport is severely restricted. Creating a training program that includes conditioning extensibility is dependent on the demands of the sport. There is a baseline of healthy extensibility all athletes need to limit injury, yet, the extent of the need is highly dependent on the type of sport the athlete is involved in. For instance, a gymnast requires full agile and extensive mobility. Whereas an MMA fighter needs less. The needs of the training coincide with the demands of the sport and the areas of development required in the athlete. The sweet spot. The triad sweet spot. It's in every type of training stimulus.

BALANCE & MOTOR CONTROL TRAINING

Fluidity of movement is predicated on balance and motor control. While the brain is highly involved in developing the blueprint to express this process, the balance systems are the extensions of that expression. When we see an athlete pristine and moving with ease through complex power and mobility, much like the baseball pitcher winding in extensive mobility and releasing a fast pitch in powerful velocity, it is the developments in the brain processing centers that make those movements possible and precise. Much of what is required in specific, complex balance and motor control movements is developed in sport specific seasons of training. Motor control is the motor memory built with repetition of practice. Balance, specific to sport, is best built in the context of that sport. It serves both to build inherent balance as well as create extensive motor memory. Building motor memory helps an athlete move through the sport with ease, allowing the mind to focus elsewhere as the body has mastered the memory of movement specific to the demand of the sport. This frees the mind up for decisive and real time interaction. An athlete needs clear headspace to engage in sport. Sport is not a mindless interaction. It is bold, decisive interaction. A fully engaged champ is a force to be reckoned with. That's the point of sport!

METABOLIC TRAINING

Stamina, endurance, power and an ability to flow between all three in a given sport is developed with metabolic training. Complex systems within our body develop and harness the stored energy from our nutrition intake to fuel the exertion a sport demands. ***Nutrition is crucial to metabolic development and training***. A soccer player shifting from one speed to another, cutting and turning on a moment's decision, racing down the end of the field toward the goal is a prime example of switching and flowing between systems. Some sports demand a mix of power and endurance, others land in any one extreme predominantly. The flow between the varying systems is conditioned with specific training. The metabolic training is the most specific type of training in regard to sport and training program design. An athlete's sport is what defines the conditioning parameters in metabolic training.

RECOVERY IN TRAINING

Recovery/rest is the other side of the training regimen. Stimulus in training engages the body, stretches its capacity and turns athletic systems on. Recovery, on the flip side, rebuilds, reorganizes, takes in the "sensation" of the stimulus internally at the deep athletic system operations and then it begins developing its ability to meet the demand with less effort.

The challenge of training is the stimulus to create change or adaptation in the body. That stimulus is the training impact while recovery builds the training effect. Do you see why it is valuable to respect the recovery? I have heard many trainers and coaches using the phrase "train smart" and it is this phrase that comes to mind when I think of the interplay between stimulus and recovery in training. It certainly is not wise to short-change the recovery and lose the benefit of the work done in the stimulus. Reaping the reward. It is here that the reward is developed.

TRAINING EFFECTS - RECOVERY

Training effect is expressed during recovery. What are the training effects? Training effects are adaptations! They occur centrally, at the heart and lungs, as well as peripherally, at the blood flow and muscle cells. There is an effect at the brain as well. Remember that the brain is the driver of systems operations. And it is this driver that integrates systems. What is peak performance? It is systems integration. The brain, central body and peripheral body adaptations are what we will discuss next.

BRAIN ADAPTATIONS

The two sides of the brain functioning together are the creative and the task completion. Think of it like this. The body acts and the body builds. Same with the brain. It instructs the body to act and it instructs the body to build. Autonomic nervous system functioning drives these two acting and building mechanisms. The sympathetic face emerging to produce movement and the parasympathetic face retreating the body into recovery and building.

In addition to this, the brain is developed emotionally. Where there is progress and development in athletic abilities, there is also progress and development in encouragement. This is the psychological phenomenon of building momentum. Momentum feeds motivation. Motivation is needed to stay in the training regimen and finish the difficult and continuously progressive tasks to completion.

Specifically in recovery, the brain pulls the body into its parasympathetic face. This command center fires up the digestive processes and is a reason recovery nutrition is so crucial. The nutrition serves to energize the building and adaptation processes in the body as well as restore the energy reserve for the next challenge. This nervous system input places the body in a state of rest, slowing the heart rate and breathing rate, bringing the visual sensation into low intensity, shunting more of the blood from the limbs and into the central parts of the body to focus the body's energy on retrieving energy and restoring the body to a state of homeostasis. The brain processes the experience, the body taking in the experience as a memory at the brain and at the cellular level. It now becomes a part of the body and a new normal, a new homeostasis is achieved. Just as much as what we eat becomes a part of who we become, so does what we experience. There is an effect, a training effect. Our body adapts to the experience both psychologically and physically. The emotion brain processes the experience and the parasympathetic system moves the body into recovering and resting adaptations.

CENTRAL BODY ADAPTATIONS

At the center of the body, the heart, our breathing capacity and the blood flow between the two is also developed. The effect of training causes efficiency. At the center of our body, that efficiency creates more power in the heart muscle with each beat. Blood shunting from the right contracting force of the heart into the lungs and from the left contracting force into the limbs. With each increase in contraction power, more blood is ejected causing the heart to beat at a quieter tempo when conditioned. Entering the lungs, more blood is available for the exchange of respiratory gases. The depth of the lungs build, expanding with greater ease. This expansion opening more lung components and improving the efficiency of air flow and exchange. As the lungs are conditioned to do more with each breath, the exchange between the blood flowing from the heart, that of carbon dioxide leaving the blood and entering our exhalation breath and oxygen entering the blood from our inhalation, becomes more efficient. What does this mean? It means more is done in each exchange than what was previously done. The effect of training is creating efficient work. The body is adapting. The same with the left contracting force of the heart. As the blood capacity of oxygen increases and it flows back into the left heart, it is pumped into the limbs with more blood being ejected in each beat. Efficiency. More with less effort. This is the training effect. The body does more with less. The quality of the work doubles. The body not only works hard at a fast pace, it also builds quality and greater impact in each progressive effort due to training. Training builds efficiency, quality and improved impact. That training effect is built in recovery.

PERIPHERAL BODY ADAPTATIONS

At the limbs, in the periphery of the body, muscle cells and metabolic energy processes receive the blood from the heart. Blood flow circulates at the cellular interface of the muscles and gas exchange occurs. The increased carrying capacity of the blood shifts more oxygen into this exchange. Efficiency in transferring the gases improves. More oxygen gets into the cell and more carbon dioxide pulls out of the cell. Oxygen feeds energy production and carbon dioxide is the cellular waste of energy production. Becoming efficient in this exchange keeps the metabolic system from being clogged with waste. The steady exchange keeps the system clean and ready for engagement.

Another cellular mechanism that becomes more efficient is the nutritional substrate retrieval. The retrieval of food energy stored in the body. This retrieval is achieved by the hormonal system, which is activated by the parasympathetic nervous system. It is the face of the parasympathetic that ignites and switches on the hormonal cascade. The series of hormones become efficient in activating the release and shunting them to the cells when the body is in a training challenge. The more energy available, the stronger the body's response to the challenge.

With each experience of training, the memory of that experience is processed in the body. It becomes a part of the body and, in essence, the body makes room for it by adapting to it. In addition to adapting the energy retrieval aspect of the periphery, the body also improves its waste removal. The cellular waste is processed at the cells with carbon dioxide shifting out more efficiently as blood flows nearby. That carbon dioxide as well as nutritional waste product is shifted into the blood to clean out the cell. The carbon dioxide travels to the lungs and is exhaled in our breath. The nutritional waste travels to the liver, is processed and broken down through a series of biochemical reactions. The neat thing about our body is its internal ability to recreate substances. It takes some metabolic byproducts, wastes, and reformulates them into substrates for energy!

THE RHYTHMS OF THE OCEAN

Approaching the water's edge, looking at the ripples and movements, feeling the cool air breeze past, she steps in. It's cooler today. Moving forward, and then stopping to give her body a moment to adjust as the wave break crashes past her.

Moving further, half immersed, diving in, hands breaking the surface and rush of cool water surrounding her arms and head afresh. The coolness rippling through her senses, the chill giving way, body feeling warm again. Surfacing in the line the wave is breaking, the force of the water erupting all around her. Diving forward, turning and surfacing on her back, afloat, lying there, suspended. Timeless. Everything seems timeless here. The ocean, wrapping itself around and surrounding her like the hug of a good friend, carrying away the stresses of life. The memory of even her body's movements fade. It's the rhythm of the wave that she is aware of. It's moving her, gracefully shifting and lifting. Unaware of where the next wave is, simply flowing with the energy as it comes. Trust. Trusting the rhythmic movement of the water. Listening to the sound, feeling the energy in the water as it builds and releases around her. Catching the rhythm and moving with it. It's like the breathing in and out of her lungs. One part active, the other passive. The energy building around her and then releasing with a ripple effect.

Remember, sports and training are really about relationship. Relationship is about trust. Trust the process. Learn to let go and trust the inherent intelligence housed within the body. When the champ is being built within, during the process of rest and recovery, there is no external effort. Only replenishment and rest. Allow the body to build. Let the involuntary work of adaptation do its work. It's time for the champ to rest. Rest and trust. This is not your time to engage! Let go. Flow. You'll have your opportunity to rise again very soon.

THE BUOYANCY OF THE SEA - THE LIFT OF RECOVERY

Floating, her mind drifts to the weightlessness of her body. It's internal sea mirroring the external sea. The effects of gravity lifted. A new force acting on her body. Bouyancy. It's the opposite of gravity. Instead of forces that press her down to the surface, keeping her grounded, it's the force of the lift. Is it healing to have a change of pace? Is it healing to be lifted rather than weighted? Is it restful to be suspended?

Recovery in training is a weightless moment on the body. It is a moment that the exertion and action is lifted. The inner resources work in our bodies, restoring, healing, lifting the burden of demand. All the while, working internally to elevate the ability within. Adapting, harnessing, developing, growing. Strengthening the body to engage the demand again. Here, again, we have yin and yang of two faces in our bodies. The face of stillness and the face of action. The rhythm of buoyancy and the effect of gravity. The lift and the stand. The energy replenishment and the energy expenditure. The rest and the demand.

Do we see that our body functions naturally in rhythms? Do we see that each rhythm has the power to do something so different than the other? There is more to recovery in a training regimen than we understand. Even without full understanding, there is more reason to appreciate it, respect it and engage in it wisely. While it is the moment of stillness in our bodies, our body is not still but highly active in functions that cannot be done otherwise. Respecting its operations is understanding the involuntary work being done behind the scenes and allowing our energy to shift to that process by adequately resting until the work is complete.

FROM CHALLENGE TO RECOVERY

Coming full circle, training for efficiency in athletic systems is a progressive and repeat process. Both the training challenge and the training recovery serves to elevate athletic ability. Although both phases of training are quite different, development is not possible without both. There is a cause and effect relationship. The training challenge causing the effect of adaptation, realized in recovery, is the point of intelligent training. Coming into alignment with the intelligence housed within our body is a win win! It is constructive growth and development. The yin and yang of which matches the rhythm of the two faces of peak performance. Turn the page and let's dive into the body's intelligence further.

CHAPTER FOUR

WHAT ABOUT THE BRAIN'S INVOLVEMENT?

H ave you ever looked into the eyes of a champion? The flame present in the eye is something caught more than seen. It's there, impacting and power-ful. The passion burning bright, the culture within creating a sense about the person. We sense it, take it in, experience it, even though we cannot see it, touch it, look directly at it. It's there though. Carrying presence and lifting the soul of our humanity as we witness it. Inspiring us, calling out greatness within. They say the eyes are the window to the soul.

The soul of a champion, the heart of a champion, brings life to a body. Birthing strength, power, endurance and overcoming stamina in the face of great challenge. Consistently rising to meet the challenge is the defining overture of a champion. Facing them over and over, developing and rising internally as they consistently rise and step forward to meet the demand head on. Powerfully engaging the challenge, the champion is built from the inside out. Rising internally to rise externally, the depths of training building the heights of strength and power.

Housed beyond the eyes of a well built athlete is the soul. The emotion brain. Motivating and lifting, the soul empowers the body. Constructive and healthy, the emotion brain adds its weight to the game and participates in the heavy lift of sport engagement. Reaching the heights of peak performance without a healthy soul is much like running on a shifting surface, dribbling a deflated basketball or playing tennis without a net. Something is missing. A crucial piece. Missing this piece undermines an athlete's capabilities. Bringing life to the soul brings life to the body. It brings life to the game. What is sport other than an interaction of a fully alive individual, impacting and engaging with a force of energy that is vibrant, real and powerful?

The opposite of life is a draining, burn out. Think about those words. Burn out. The flame is burnt out. The flame representing a fully alive, vibrant and engaged athlete. With burn out, the alive and passionate engagement within an athlete dies. A burned out soul is a soul on the brink of death. Burnout is the soul injured and deflated within. It is the overworked athlete, tanked in motivation and detoured from the finish line. What follows this other than a loss of confidence, a loss of stamina, a loss of emotional strength? The emotion brain is the seat of our emotional strength, mental strength and psychological stamina in the face of challenge and difficulty. Sadly, it can burn out and respecting that line allows the athlete to protect their soul as much as protecting their physical abilities. Have you ever seen a champion with a burned out soul? Have you ever seen a victory lap done with deflation or resignation? Have you ever seen a champ standing on a podium to receive a reward with shoulders slumped and disappointment shattering their nonverbal expressions? Of course not.

The emotion brain is just as important as the thinking brain. It's the juice behind the kick. No juice, no kick. It packs a power that ignites the physical. The roar of that inner giant, releasing its guttural and wild call. Free to energize, free to soar. It rides high, elevating every physical effort. Pain isn't as noticeable. The pain of the stretch likened to a friend instead of a foe. The emotion brain releasing powerful endorphins, lifting the body above the discomfort of discipline and training, adding a joyous element to it all. Did you ever notice that a broken heart causes everything to feel painful? Why does a broken spirit, a discouraged heart cower? The emotion brain is dismantled.

The body weakens. It is heavily influenced by the emotion brain.

Building mental strength does not require a slip into destructive emotional constructs. The delicate balance of a healthy emotion brain is impacted by respecting its limits and remaining constructive in its exertions. If it is heavily influenced in the negative emotional construct, how much more will it soar when influenced in a healthy emotional construct and manner?

Resonance. Bringing the peak out of athletes requires building a constructive foundation. Construction is the act of building. Destruction is the act of tearing down. The emotion brain is the delineating line between relational construction and destruction. That relating directly affects confidence, belief and courage. Breaking confidence in an athlete is a sabotaging effort. ***The point of peak performance is to build both athletic competence and confidence.***

That sweet and healthy integration between the emotion brain and the thinking brain brings competence and confidence into alignment with one another. Powerful athletes carry a presence in the game. That is confidence. Without it, competence has no outlet. Without the emotion brain, the thinking brain has no outlet because it is the emotion brain that causes the athlete to show up to the game and engage. Building both is what creates powerful athletes!

The emotion brain is also as important as the sensing brain, and the acting brain. What good is it to be motivated to move and know how to competently engage if the ability to sense and act in the sport interaction is disabled? One must be able to feel the impact in the game as well as produce the physical expression of the brain's decision to impact. In the brain, those two areas comprise the sensing and acting operations. The sensory and motor processing are the hands and feet of the brain, so to speak.

There really are four broad aspects to the brain: the emotion brain, thinking brain, sensing brain and acting brain. Emotional, social and relational, the emotion brain contributes to the quality of life. The emotion brain is like the interior decorator of a house. The structure is robotic and lifeless without it. Coming to life and creating the feel of a home is what interior design is meant to do. Much like the interior designer in a home, the emotion brain adds the cultural feel and presence to a home. Logical, reasonable, comprehensible, intuitive and analytical, the thinking brain develops order and organizes thoughts, attitudes and actions. The sensing brain receives and processes our world and the acting brain acts on our world.

Each aspect of the brain plays a separate role and yet, influences one another. Complex integration and organization either builds or dismantles the functioning of our brain. Twisted and chaotic, dissonant and destructive at any point or in any part, the brain becomes dysfunctional. In some ways, it even becomes diseased. It is a lack of ease, a lack of harmony, a lack of resonance. When in harmony, resonance is built from within. Health is creating an integration in the brain that serves the purpose of constructive growth. Layer upon layer, the effort in all areas build alongside one another. Connections interweaving and health flowing freely in all directions, the brain's function is elevated and peak performance is harnessed.

THE POWER OF INTERACTION IS IN THE BRAIN

The brain, the center of our body's ability to sense and receive, act and engage, recover and rebuild, defines the art of interaction. Interaction happens as the brain senses its surroundings, processes that information, integrates that understanding with other parts of the brain, makes decisions and then acts on that decision. The brain is where interaction happens. The body is where it is sensed and expressed.

Standing authentic and strong, the development of who we are, what we stand for, the unique characteristics, the passion and inherent interests that make us distinct from those around us, we stand defined by our development. Developed and yet ever growing, changing and adapting as we interact. Impacting and being impacted. The interactions of life touching us as we touch life all around us. While the substance and power behind our impact is worked out in our brain, it is the brain that drives our interactions in life. Building interaction, creating presence and engaging with the surroundings is what brings our body to life. It is what brings life to our interactions as well.

THE MAIN PLAYER IN SPORT INTERACTION IS THE BRAIN

Building interaction in sport through play, through the play of a structured game, is what athletes enjoy. They love the game. They love the interaction of challenge. What is play but the authentic and powerfully engaged presence of one player interacting with that of another? Play is the interaction in the game of sport. That interactive power, the ability to experience and engage, rests in the mechanisms of the brain. Sport provides an opportunity for our brain to reveal its substance and authenticity. It is also an opportunity to develop and grow by the impact of sport and training. We are sharpened as the edge of our ability is tested and stretched over and over. Some say "iron sharpens iron" and perhaps this applies as the strength and power of one player tests the limits of another player, sharpening and fine-tuning one another in the challenge.

That sharpening, the physical expression of it before the eyes of spectators and coaches and trainers and onlookers alike, represents a deeper sharpening. So many systems involved, the main power of all those systems being the brain. Impacting the body to impact the sport, the brain fires up and electrically ignites the body through nerve impulse. Every organ system expressed in athletic expression is ignited by the electrical power in the brain. It begins and ends in the brain. The full circle of interaction and, in this case, the full circle of sport interaction is housed within our phenomenal, mysterious, deeply studied and still not completely conquered brain. What is the brain's involvement with peak performance? What is the brain's involvement with sport interaction? What is the brain's involvement with training? Everything. It touches everything. Everything touches it. It is the beginning and the end. The center of it all. It is the seat of interaction. Do you see that yet?

Impacting and being impacted. The sport serving to supply the stage for the power in the brain to display its excellence, its development, its magnificence. The athletically fit brain is developed, strong and deeply coordinated. It is brain fit. We tend to look at athletes and judge their athleticism by their outward appearance, which does help absolutely. It's an interesting thought to wonder what the fit brain looks like! While assessing its outward appearance is not possible like that of, for example, muscle strength, the expression of that outward appearance is displayed through the movements of the body.

The finely tuned athlete that moves with ease through complex movement patterns is brain fit. Combining velocity, force trajectory, angle of movement, whole body integration versus deeply controlled peripheral movements are just a few examples of a highly trained and fit brain. The more complex the movements a sport demands, with the more interactive elements and spontaneous changes within the sport interaction, the more brain fitness is demanded. The brain is highly engaged with complexity. Layers of complexity come into play at all levels of brain function when a game challenges an athlete in a complex manner.

THE POWER OF IMPACT

The brain is a complex organization. It is the command of our actions, the feeler of our body, the processor of our thoughts, sensation and actions, and our inherent memory. While we live in a world that acts upon us, our mind is, in itself, an action upon the world. It is where the world is imprinted upon us and where the will within imprints our presence on our world. Our bodies would be dead bones and debilitated muscles without the brain. The brain brings life to the body. It brings direction and is the source of our personhood that interacts with our world.

Within this complex organization of our brain, the thinking and emotion aspect of it create widely different results and effects in our body. While these effects are different, they have the potential to build on one another. Unfortunately, they also have the potential to work against one another. They create impact and, at the same time, are impacted.

IMPACT IS ENERGY TRANSFER

Impact is the work of an athlete in their sport. Remember that an athlete releases energy onto the context of their sport and that energy is rebounded back to them. This is the interactive process of sport. The greater the impact, the greater the development. Impact is the work. Work is the transfer of movement energy onto another object or surface.

When a soccer ball is moved by the powerful energy in the foot of Mia Hamm, the energy is transferred from her foot and into the ball, sending it onto a trajectory. The more precision and power behind that development, the more energy transferred. What is athletics other than the force of an athletic presence impacting their sport like a prevailing force? What is a champion other than a powerful force? What is a champion other than an impact? When she shows up, things change. The force of her presence requires a shift in the game.

THE EXCHANGE OF IMPACT IS FELT IN THE BRAIN

In full speed, legs pumping forward. One and then the other. The ball volleying along with her, passing effortlessly between her feet. Her eyes engaging her target. Peripheral vision taking in what is around her, scanning the visual field for defensive movements. Brain calculating the distance, synapse of electrical impulse carrying her visual intake to the processing centers of her brain. Within milliseconds, the processing translating into quick decisive action. Decision made. Electric impulses commanding her body to prepare her winning move. Body slows. She sees her moment. Placing the ball a few feet in front of her, widening her stride. Moving in with body winding in counter force, lengthening. She's there. Pulling everything to her center, powerfully and explosively carrying her body through, the inside of her foot making contact with the ball. Not stopping there, the follow through continues as the ball lands in the net, just beyond the reach of her opponent's hands. The winning move. Made. Teammates rushing in at her. Excitement pumping through the air. Bodies exploding with expressions of victory and excitement, unable to be contained. The power of the thinking brain just impacted the emotion brain. Mia Hamm.

INTEGRATED EMOTION AND THINKING BRAIN

The neuropsychology aspect of the human body is what I will refer to as the connection between our emotion brain and the executive decision making in our actions, the thinking brain. The emotion brain is the interaction in the brain between the prefrontal cortex and the limbic system. The limbic system is the seat of our emotions and the motivations of our actions. It is the affective component of our humanity. I like to think of it as the culture of our existence. In general terms, we tend to think of this aspect of our brain as the "heart" attitudes and attributes in our lives. The affective components are inclusive of the why and the how in the five ways we process our lives. They are the "why" and "how" in the carrying out of the "what", "when" and "where" logistics in our thinking brain processing. The emotion brain creates the culture behind the actions. The thinking, cognitive brain focuses on the technical aspects of life - the what, when and where. But, it's the emotion brain that gives those aspects meaning and context and thus, creates the culture in which those operate and exist.

IS EMOTIONAL INTELLIGENCE RELEVANT?

Taking it one step further, the emotion brain is where our emotional intelligence is developed. The cognitive brain is where our intelligence quotient is developed. Both processes of learning are vastly different.

Primitive emotional intelligence, or undeveloped emotion brain function leads to inability to feel empathy, create relational connections, inability to be self-aware, inability to be socially aware, and lacking in constructive emotional motivations. These deficits create what is referred to as "dissonance" in relationships. This is a deeper divide between people and people groups. Instead of creating greater community, individuals that have not developed emotional intelligence quotients tend to marginalize communities and create toxic environments as they perpetuate dysfunctional emotional constructs as the driver and motivator of their actions. When these negative thought and emotion constructs drive actions, it perpetuates in an individual's relationships and reduces their ability to develop self confidence and perform at their peak. We are, by nature, social creatures and the people we surround ourselves with have a profound influence on how we think, behave and relate to ourselves as well as to others. We are impacted by their presence. There is a phenomenon called "limbic locking" that speaks to this very thing. Limbic locking is the influence that occurs in groups when a leader begins to perpetuate actions from their emotion brain. It is the attunement of the crowd to what is perpetuating in the group. The limbic systems of the individuals surrounding a strong personality will begin to catch the culture that is created from that person's limbic system. "More is caught than taught" is a phrase that makes sense in the limbic locking phenomenon.

The emotion brain is initially developed from birth up to our twenties, with its basic foundation of experience, nurturing and development. Of course, we know that growth of any aspect of our human bodies occurs as a mix between genetics and nurture. It is the nature versus nurture in unison played out in our growth process. The formative years, of course, lay down our "default" foundation. These are the "go to" reactions, or put another way, the habits, the unconscious and subconscious ways in which we respond in situations. Once we are beyond our twentieth year, in order to undo the foundation, there is a lengthy process we must undergo. It requires intentional work, repetition and dedication because it is what is required to undo the old and replace it with the new. If the supports were not present, internally and externally in terms of genetics or a nurturing growth environment, these can be recovered. The learning in the emotion brain is different than the learning in the cognitive brain; it is lengthier and requires more wisdom application, outside feedback from peers and mentors and practice for growth. But, it can be done. Our brains are neuroplastic and that includes the emotion brain.

There is one side of the brain in the prefrontal cortex and limbic connection that produces nerve impulses when emotional intelligence is highly developed. The other side is predominant when it is rudimentary and under-developed. These skills are crucial for peak performance because constructive and healthy relationship to one's self as well as to the community create an atmosphere and culture of resonance. Resonance produces an energized productivity. Meaning, the work load with resonance actually energizes rather than depletes an individual. It creates more good will, motivation and drive with energy expenditure. Whereas dissonance, which is associated with low emotional intelligence, creates a depletion of energy from work. It is psychologically taxing and exhausting rather than up-lifting. This is very important to the principles of burnout psychologically, cognitively and physically. Peak performance remains in the therapeutic zone of productivity and the sweet spot of energy expenditure that produces even more energy. In everyday type of language, it would be the difference between flying with the eagles mentality with high vision and squawking with the turkeys over the scraps. It's the culture of the mind that transcends destructive emotions that tend to tear down a group and create self-destructive tendencies within an individual. One cannot build on a foundation that is being undermined by one's own destructive emotion. ***Harnessing peak performance is developing a healthy emotional intelligence.***

PROCESSING IMPACT

The neurocognitive brain is the portion of our brains that make executive decisions. It is the area where we decide how our bodies will move as we process the input our sensory system has given to us about our environments. It is largely present in the prefrontal cortex of our brain. This is the frontal lobe area and its name assists us in locating where it is in the brain - it is in the front, located directly behind our foreheads.

The cognitive functions of our brain include working memory, learning, communication, decision-making, processing all of our incoming sensory information, such as vision, hearing, balance, proprioception and touch, and deciding what to do with it. It is the "what, where, when" of our processing. The logic and reason of our brains. The sensory system is our relationship to our environment. It gives the brain information about it's location in space through joint proprioceptors; muscle length through muscle spindle fibers; tendon stretch through Golgi tendon organs; touch and vibration sensation through our skin receptors; and visual field information, vestibular/balance and head position through our inner ear organ. This information is received in the parietal lobe, temporal lobe and occipital lobe. The primary somatosensory area has an internal map that lights up to specific areas for sensation. The adjacent somatosensory association area processes that information in more detail. This information is then bounced around to the basal ganglia nuclei for motor planning, sequencing of movement and regulating movement force and tone. Communication loops bounce between primary motor cortex, the basal ganglia and the premotor cortex for deep processing, decision-making and motor execution. Electrical impulse extends down from the basal ganglia and into the brainstem through the pyramidal tracts. Some shoot over to the cerebellum at the pons for feedforward cerebellar actions and further precision of movement prior to continuing down to the spinal cord and out the corresponding level to extend through a peripheral nerve and complete the actions.

Vision and balance are processed through special sense organs. Vision is processed through our eyes, the optic nerve and then at the corresponding nuclei. The information is sent to the occipital lobe of the brain for further processing at the vision centers. That information is attained at the association areas, which are really areas of higher brain functions and processing. That communication is shared and used to bring more input into movement and executive decisions.

Balance is processed through our inner ear organ where particles shift depending on our head position, telling our body where our head is relative to gravity. Did you notice how your vision remains the same no matter what position you place your head? That is a result of the VOR reflex (vestibulo-ocular reflex) that works to maintain our visual field while we tilt and move our head. If this doesn't prove that the world does not revolve around a human, it might be wise to ask why this internal perspective - righting system exists in us, keeping the world steady as we revolve around it. Asking why gravity works to anchor us to the earth's surface rather than the earth being anchored to us is another good question. On a comical note, it would be a little chaotic if it was reversed. Think about it. How many people are on the planet? Can you imagine the earth trying to revolve around each of us individually? That would be chaos and disorder. Digression.

The visual system is a powerful sensory organ. What is the purpose of sensory organs? How do they assist athletes in their sport? Our sensory system gives us information about what we are acting on, our environment. For the athlete, that becomes their sport surface. An opponent, a ball or some type of surface is what an athlete interacts with while engaging in their sport. It is important for them to see, feel, hear, smell and taste to engage with what is around them. In athletics, the sensation of taste is likely not involved much. Unless you are in a corndog eating contest during a basketball tournament, learning the art of mowing down while dribbling around an opponent. Well, that would be unlikely as the two actions engage opposing autonomic nervous system functions. It would be a serious internal conflict, felt heavily in the gut of your inner knower. Don't advise it. Not compatible. Divorce that idea now, it's an inevitable contradiction, k.

The sensory systems involved with athletics are mostly vision, hearing, proprioception and touch sensations. These systems give data to our brain for cognitive and emotional processing. Our cognitive brain orders it, makes sense of it and decides what, if anything, to do with it. Our emotion brain stores a working memory with the experience, creating an emotional association with an event. Once the brain has processed this input, the rest of the body carries out the decisions the brain has made with that information.

The visual system, in this scenario, serves to provide executive decision making in real time, provide insight to your balance system and body awareness.

SPECIAL SENSES

There are a number of special senses that contribute to movement in the neuromuscular system. These include the visual, the vestibular, the somatic sensory and postural. These three special senses combine to form our balance reactions as well as planning our movements. They combine their sensory input to provide both reactive and proactive movements. Both are needed. For instance, the reactive movement strategies are important in sports like surfing, where the surface is spontaneously creating movement and ground reaction forces under the athlete. Meaning, the surface is changing in real time and it is not possible to see every change coming prior to dealing with that change. So, in surfing, the ability to react using these three balance systems is crucial to a person's ability to handle the dynamics of surfing. In contrast, the sport of downhill skiing has a fixed surface. The surface does not change much and an athlete is able to plan their movement mechanics in advance of the time the movement is needed.

The visual system uses our eyes as a sense organ to give our minds information about the environment, surface or obstacle we are acting on in a sport. The vestibular system is a sense organ within our inner ear that gives our brains our position in space. It also orients our visual field to maintain its position regardless of whether our head turns, tilts or if we are standing on our hands in an inverted position. It functions to keep our visual field consistent no matter what position our head ends up being in!

The somatosensory system, especially in our feet, helps us feel what surface we are standing on as well as provides positional information from our joints. These positional senses are our proprioceptors and are located in joints. They tell us where they are in space when we are not looking. It basically gives our brain a map of each part of our body at all times. Close your eyes, take your finger and touch your nose. Notice that you did that without actively looking to find your finger and guiding it to your nose visually. This activity was able to be done because you relied on your internal body map, the proprioceptors that create an image map in your brain.

With all three systems operating and providing information to our brain, our brain is then able to motor plan. Motor planning is a proactive planning of our movements in anticipation of an action that will need to be taken. It is a part of a communication loop that takes the sensory information and processes it in our cerebellum (the back end of our brain) and then creates postural adjustments, changes in movements and balance actions in an anticipation of future movements. The reactive movement mechanisms are planned in real time, are quick, decisive and immediate. The sensory information is processed at the spinal level, at the brain level and then reactions are created from the spinal level and the cerebellum in a feedback loop. So, training for a specific sport requires an analysis of the biomechanics of the sport and a strategic, intelligent matching of the training to enhance the athlete's systems that are primarily engaged in the sport.

In a conversation I had with a friend last year, he mentioned his frustration over being able to snowboard without a problem but having difficulty with surfing. He was frustrated because the movements seemed similar. Yet, the one thing that is often missed in training is assessing the surface the movements are occurring on. And in both of these sports, the surfaces were radically different. One was stable, unmoving and the other was a dynamic force that developed with a general pattern but with random, spontaneous ground reaction forces that developed under the board. In both of these sports, there was a similarity in the athletic movements but there was a very discrete difference between the balance system's engagement, the use of sensory information in the brain and the neural pathways that responded in action. This certainly highlighted that similar movements could look a lot alike but use very different parts of the brain for processing. In my friends case, he was efficient in the feedforward and motor planning mechanisms in snowboarding, yet his body experienced a challenge, not because he was not capable, but because he was now being challenged in a feedback motor reaction as well as placing his body in an environment that required consistent and sporadic spontaneous balance adjustments in the surfing. Truly, the sporting demand of surfing, while it looks similar, is quite different than snowboarding!

MOTOR LEARNING

The training primes our bodies to create responses that become automatic, much like what happens when we learn how to ride a bike. This is called motor learning in brain science language. It is the process of teaching our bodies a movement task by breaking it down to its parts and then integrating the parts back into the whole. In the end, what was quite difficult at first becomes much like "learning to ride a bike" and thereafter, not much thought is put into the task due to the development of motor planning and learning with this movement. Initially, the process of learning to ride a bike takes an inordinate amount of time and each task must be broken down to its most basic form. Slowly, each piece is learned and then integrated. What began as a very conscious effort and laborious thought process becomes automatic, a task that one now seems to be able to do without much direct thought. In fact, one is now able to focus on other tasks and multi-task on top of this once complicated and difficult task. This is the art of motor learning. It is important to specificity of training for any sport movement and it is an aspect of the brain's function in producing defined and skilled movements.

The result of motor learning is highly developed movement patterns. Shifting from high level of attention to task to an automatic pattern of movement, movement patterns become fine-tuned. The area involved in developing this ease of movement is the deep part of the brain called the basal ganglia. There are other areas involved but this area is where movements become fine tuned and where they become a part of who we are so much so that it is where we "rely on our instincts" during our athletic games. We hear this often. When it is game time, we are told to let go and rely on the training. What we are really saying is "trust the training process in our basal ganglia". When we have conditioned ourselves over and over in a movement, as we do in specificity of training, that neuropathway within the movement circuitry of our brain, inclusive of the basal ganglia, become so deeply ingrained that the conscious effort is no longer needed. It is learned, habitual and much more automatic. It is "fine-tuned". The beauty of a fine tuned athlete, pristine in movement, effortless in expression. That is the intelligent work of our basal ganglia. There is another area that plays into this work. The cerebellum. Both the basal ganglia and cerebellum take basic movement patterns and add fine adjustments, causing them to appear refined and artistic. Is that not what athletic expression is? Is that not why we watch athletics so deeply?

FEEDFORWARD AND FEEDBACK ADJUSTMENTS

In the cerebellum, our brains also take in information from our body's sense of awareness in space (proprioception) to

136

give us feedback on our balance in movement patterns. It does this proactively and retroactively through neural connections at the spinal level and cerebellar level. Movement is not solely musculoskeletal. It is profoundly neuromuscular and the neuromuscular component is even more important in specificity of movement than the musculoskeletal aspect. When we are looking to create highly specific movement patterns, it is motor learning, motor planning, cognitive decision making and feedback/feedforward adjustments that provide the fine details and help train our bodies to create seemingly effortless and automatic movement patterns. While this is an incredible aspect to our bodies, it is also one to proceed with extreme caution in. This is where bad habits are developed and become extremely difficult to break so shortcuts in training will create deep cracks in the foundation of all that work. It is wise to build steadily, intelligently and carefully because what is built through motor learning is very difficult to unlearn. Yet, when it is built correctly, there is a return on that investment that becomes highly rewarding in the athletic abilities attained.

NEUROENDOCRINE SYSTEM

The neuroendocrine system begins at the HPA axis, which is an abbreviation for hypothalamic-pituitary adrenal axis. The HPA axis is what modulates and primes our bodies for adaptation to stress and strain in our bodies. It's what is activated when our bodies go into an intense mode of operation.

This system is the intersection of the autonomic nervous system and the hormonal systems. It is important to the hormonal cascades that drive communication through the body's various systems and functions. You might be thinking, what is a hormonal cascade? It is one hormone being released into the blood stream or into an organ as a result of another hormone activating its release. Think of it like playing a game of "tag", or perhaps, in athletic lingo, think of it as the baton hand-off of an athlete finishing their 100 meter part in a 400 meter dash race. In the body, each piece plays a part in the bigger vision of its collective organization.

In general, both the hormonal system and nervous system serve as the communication drivers in the body. They connect as well as integrate the functions of our body's many systems. They drive that communication from the nervous system input. Remember, our brain is the decision-maker and ultimate driver of our actions, both conscious and unconscious. It's the command center and source of electrical power, sent out to the remaining parts of our body. Although, now we are learning that the components of each system of the body have more interdependence that what we originally knew. Meaning, there is more inherent functioning within each system.

The nervous system charges our body, including our hormones into communicating the brain's commands. The nervous system also receives insights and understanding about the environment from the body and utilizes that to influence decisions of how to relate. So, let's turn back to the neuroendocrine component of this discussion.

The neuroendocrine system is kick-started by the hypothalamus aspect of the brain, where nerve tissue is then extended into the posterior pituitary. For a quick review, the nervous system part of the neuroendocrine system is the hypothalamus of the brain and it is in the deep center of the brain, above the brainstem. Connected to the hypothalamus are some hormonal structures (also called endocrine system components). These structures are the pituitary glands, which sit in front of the hypothalamus and each have two parts: the anterior and posterior pituitary gland. The pineal gland is another endocrine component and it sits behind the hypothalamus. The pineal gland is not a part of the HPA axis but I thought I would mention it here because of its close association to the hypothalamus.

So, we are back to the HPA axis. What is the purpose of the nervous tissue extensions of the hypothalamus? Remember that the hypothalamus is brain tissue, and in case we didn't clarify earlier, brain tissue is nerve tissue. Basically the brain is a large mass of nervous and electrical conduction! Power source. So, here we are with the pituitary gland sitting right next to the hypothalamus. The hypothalamus sends nerve endings into the gland, specifically the posterior pituitary, and there it controls the manufacturing and release of hormones that either suppress or release other hormones in the endocrine system and throughout the body.

What do hormones do, you might be asking. They communicate and turn on or suppress various functions through the organ systems. I'd say they have some of the most diverse job descriptions in the body. They function to turn on and off certain cellular functions that drive what happens in different systems. For instance, the anterior pituitary releases a number of tropic hormones. These are the "tag" or "legs of a race" style hormones, meaning their entire purpose is to activate other hormones. These type of hormones generally target organs that then release a number of other hormones. For instance, the adrenocorticotropic hormone is released from the anterior pituitary gland into the circulatory system and then targets or impacts the adrenal cortex (the outer layer) of the adrenal glands. Its presence then causes the adrenal cortex to release its hormones into the bloodstream to generally prepare the body for certain situations. The hormones released from it are mineralocorticoids (outer later of the cortex), which are the aldosterone hormones, the glucocorticoids (middle layer of the cortex), which are the cortisol hormones, and the sex hormones (inner layer of the cortex), which are the androgens.

To understand what the activation of the adrenal cortex means, we need to understand the role and purpose of the adrenal glands. The adrenal glands prepare the body for stressful circumstances. Basically, they prepare the body to create extreme physical reaction and movement. They are active in dangerous and stressful situations as well as in high level exercise. They are not designed to be active all the time and can result in exhaustion and burnout if on over-stimulation. To prepare the body for this state, these hormones target different parts of the body that play a role in this.

ACTIVATION OF PEAK PERFORMANCE

Preluding into the next section, we are going to see how the HPA axis, motor learning, the emotion brain, the cognitive brain, our hormone cascade turn our champ into an active king and then lay that champ to rest in a recovering chill zone. It's time to take a look at the two faces of peak performance.

CHAPTER FIVE

THE TWO FACES OF PEAK PERFORMANCE

Systems stepping forward, one and then the other, like two faces emerging to reveal the active champ and the resting champ. Like a toggle switch within, they ebb and flow. One explodes onto the surface, revealing the development within the champ. The other withdraws into deep processing, building the champ within. Developing. Fine-tuning. Working in tandem with one another, they generate whole body states that harness the systems into one main focus. A unified purpose as one ebbs and the other flows. Moment by moment, that purpose is either an expression of growth or development of growth. The two faces serve two different purposes, both of which serve the main vision of training up a champ in the way they should go! The path of which is laid before them, leading them intelligently along to cross the finish line of peak performance.

Like two sides to the same coin, the game face of our autonomic nervous system correlates with the two faces of exertion and rest. Our body flows between two main rhythms, that of the sleeping and resting cycle and the awake and active cycle. This cycle is not a 50/50 ratio. We spend two-thirds of our daily life awake and only one-third engaged in sleep. Within the daily wake cycle, our body fluctuates between rest and work, digestion and exertion.

Specifically, in the sport interaction, the two faces of the autonomic nervous system correlate with the two faces of training. When in the game, the champ is ignited and on, full systems engaged. With no rest for the weary until the finish line is crossed, game on means the champ is on.

THE TWO FACES OF THE CHAMP WITHIN

What are these two faces? Training includes both stimulus and recovery, we've seen that clearly now. The body's engagement in the training has two faces in that interchange.

The face of action and the face of rest. When the body is in full action mode, the face of the sympathetic nervous system is at the forefront. When the body is in the recovery and rest mode of training, the face of the parasympathetic nervous system is at the forefront. What does it mean to be at the forefront? The autonomic nervous system controls two states of the body that do not function at the same time. When one comes forward, the other pulls back. When at the forefront, that face presents itself in the athletic presence of the athlete. Athletic presence during and after. One engages the athlete in the game, the other strengthens the athlete, processing the effect of the game. There is a relationship between training stimuli and the body. Remember that a relationship creates impact. There is influence, there is interchange. The impact and influence is processed and internalized in recovery. Just like our bodies need sleep cycles, there is a rhythm of action and rest in us. That rhythm penetrates all that we do, including training.

THE ENGAGED CHAMP

The roar emerging from within, the inner champ rising, the call to the challenge igniting a response. The face of the engaged champ, primed. Ready for impact. Systems on. Electricity flowing and turning the switches on. Systems are a go, the hand of the engaged champ, the sympathetic face of action, is reaching deep into the body's inner workings. Touching and electrically igniting. Waking the body for action. Eyes engaged, open wide and deeply processing the surroundings. Hormones pumping, energizing, releasing nutrients, developing fuel flow, putting to rest the internal building processes. Harnessing energy for action. It's time to go.

With the rising roar of the engaged champ, the active champ, there is an ebb and flow. As the action and force of impact is released in the game of sport and the victory of expression complete, the champ then settles into rest and recovery.

THE RECOVERING CHAMP

Eyes turning inward, symbolically closing, focusing less, taking in less, the body is at rest. The roar quiets, the ignited release of the inner champ centers into stillness. The face of the active and engaged champ pulling back, turning off the electric energy to its systems, switching its system operations off. The body's internal sensory processing focuses on the experience. Analyzing, sequencing, replaying, organizing, experiencing, taking it all in. The impact of the interaction deeply processed. The body receiving instructions from that processing, instructions to improve and meet the challenge with a stronger interaction. "This is what we do", the body says. "Let's build, strengthen and prepare to do it again". The body, intelligently working to improve interactions and engagement. Adaptation. Flooding the body, recovering, rebuilding. With replenishment, the digestive systems light up. The inner champ laid to rest, the face of the parasympathetic system emerging. Its hand extending through the body, turning the tide of hormonal cascades, lighting up the machinery of cellular development, expansion and growth. Growth and development is its focus. The body's energy is harnessed for that one purpose at the face of the recovering champ, the face of the parasympathetic system.

THE EBB & FLOW

Peak performance training is a development of the ebb and flow between these two faces of the body. The faces, representing the two ways energy is harnessed and used during training, are symbolic of our resting and active state. Harnessing energy, the body is able to efficiently pull back some operations to prioritize others. Performing at peak capabilities requires an effective harnessing of the body's energy. It would be a chaotic and wasteful mess if every function of the body was employed at once. There are many purposes of our body and it is the mind that drives those purposes. The mind toggles the body between parasympathetic and sympathetic expression. Flowing with the two faces of the champ, the two primary systems coordinate the rhythms of our daily life, and, most notably, that which is within our athletic pursuits. Coordinating activity and rest is the ebb and flow.

As much as our body is designed to ebb and flow in a resting and active state, so much more the reason our training regimen must as well. Peak Performance Training is designed to work with the design of our bodies to improve and elevate its functioning. To train intelligently, we need to match the training methods to the natural rhythms of our body. We must train both faces of the champ: the parasympathetic/recovering champ and the sympathetic/active champ.

While training involves activity and recovery, the autonomic nervous system involves the parasympathetic nervous system (PNS) and the sympathetic nervous system (SNS). When activity is the demand, SNS steps forward and PNS steps back. When recovery is the demand, PNS steps forward and SNS steps back. As such, the nervous stimulus from the predominant system trickles through the body and prepares it. The SNS dilating the pupils to allow the visual system to take in more in the field of view and analyze deeper, increasing blood pressure to shunt blood further to muscles for activity, elevating heart rate and strength of the heart's muscular contraction to press the blood further through circulation, opening sweat glands to release the rising internal body heat, stimulating the release of hormonal cascades that prime the body for action, opening the airways into the lungs for fuller and deeper breathing. All of the SNS stimulus awakens the sleeping giant within. It awakens our inner athlete, the workhorse in us. Can we respect that the SNS is crucial?

Where does the PNS fit? It is the symbolic sleep cycle of that inner athlete, allowing the giant to rest and recover. The PNS brings our body into a state of rest, turning the attention inward, shifting the energy to a different process and slowing down our physical expression. Our pupils constrict and rest from taking in large amounts of visual sensation, calming our mind down and relaxing the executive function of our mind some while shifting its energies to adaptation mechanisms, fine-tuning processes and cleaning out cellular debris. Breathing slows, reducing the airways of the lungs. Slowing our heart rate, shunting our blood through vasoconstriction of its vessels, routing the blood resource to the inner organs for processing, replenishing and rebuilding begins. The blood floods into the digestive tract, preparing to replenish the energy stores within the body with the post exercise recovery meal. The PNS purpose of rest is to refuel, adapt, strengthen and build for the next challenge. With the lifting work of the PNS, the power in the challenge is met with the impeccable grace and poise. The development of the champ is in the flow of power and grace.

THE FLOW OF POWER & GRACE

There is a deep, settled stillness in the rhythm of the waves. Arms open, breathing deep, floating along the surface, she focuses in on the rhythm in the movement around her. Feeling the gentle touch of the water carrying her along its edge, effortlessly flowing and carrying her. All else fades into the distance, there is nothing else but her and the ocean. Connecting, learning the rhythms, her mind calms and centers its attention on the movements in the water around her and beneath her. Ebbing and flowing, ebbing and flowing. The mix of both stillness and power expressed along the ocean's edge. Allowing her senses to take it in, the awareness of its movements gracefully shifting her, moving her, lifting her. She becomes lost in the graceful dance and rhythms for a moment. Grace and power. There's grace and power in the wave. Moments of settled peace intermingled with moments of awe and respect for the powerful forces curling down off the break of the wave. Shifting her position, allowing her grace to match its grace, her power to match its power. Matching energies. Rhythms attuning. The power of resonance.

This beautiful element of the earth winning over her heart, wooing her deeper into studying its ways. As she ventures out further, there's a simultaneous calm sense of peace and a nervous energy in her. Knowing it's powerful, knowing there's still so much more to experience and learn, she pulls back. Looking out over the horizon, head above water, one last gaze. That's enough for today. The encounter closing for now. Anticipation birthing in her, her thoughts shift to the next meeting, the next encounter, the deeper connection. She steps out. This is only the beginning. The beginning of a deep relationship. Deep calling unto deep.

MANAGING THE SWEET SPOT, STAYING IN THE FLOW

Matching energies, building resonance and flowing with both power and grace, the athlete learns to experience the powerful challenge of training and the graceful lift of adaptation as her body recovers, develops and grows. This is the sweet spot of training, resonance and energy exchange. Power erupting from within in the face of challenge. The active and engaged face of the champ emerges. Grace lifting the champ from within in the face of rest and recovery. The resting and still champ, quietly allowing the work of adaptation to complete its course. Ebbing and flowing. Power and grace. Challenge and lift. Training and recovery.

HARNESSING ENERGY

To harness something means bringing it under control and focusing the use of energy into one specific purpose. For the champ, the overall purpose is peak performance. Peak performance, of course, has two faces. Within the two faces of the champ, the specific purposes ebb and flow. Harnessing the energy between these two systems is the work of the electrical impulse controlling the expression of them.

In our physical world, energy is fixed, meaning it cannot be added to or subtracted from. This is the principle of energy conservation. The energy in our world is an energy that is taken in and released in the interplay of activity and rest. In the context of athletics, energy can be increased in the athlete. The total energy in our world, however, is finite. It is not producible. It is both conserved and recycled. The total energy that exists in our world is the total energy that exists. The interactions in our world cause energy to flow, but energy is neither created nor destroyed.

In the context of sport, this is what we see playing out. The athlete releasing pent up energy in powerful displays on a sporting medium. The sport engaging with that energy and being impacted, absorbing that energy and then returning back toward the athlete in a rebounding rhythm of energy transfer.

In addition to the interplay between the athlete and the sport, there is an energy that is released from within the athlete. This is the moment the champ emerges. It is the activation of the SNS, awaking the giant within, preparing for an explosion of energy.

When the energy is released, and the athlete is exhausted, the body moves into a state of recovery and rest. The PNS takes over and lays the champ to rest, working to build new strength and adapt to overcome the challenge placed on it. The champ lays silently as the body replenishes, refuels, recovers, becomes more efficient, and builds the champ. We often think that recovery is for the weak. To shortchange the recovery is to stop the overcoming process of growth and development. It is here, in rest, that the champ is built.

ACTIVATING THE TOGGLE SWITCH

SNS/PNS activation is driven by the emotion brain at the HPA axis. Motivation shifting the body, igniting change and steering its activity. The neural input and hormone cascade trickling through like a ripple effect. Electrical impulse coursing through nerves at faster speeds than the hormones circulating in the blood stream. Both of which tempering the body, bringing it under the command of either face of the champ being stimulated at the HPA axis.

The HPA axis is the center point of where the nervous system in our brain meets our hormonal system, driving its signals into multiple systems and across all sorts of bodily functions. It has the power to cripple a person, causing them to freeze in fear. It can also cause them to fight or flee in fear. High reactivity occurs at a malfunctioning HPA axis, driven by an imbalanced limbic system, our emotion brain. A balanced emotion brain produces a balanced "active and alert body" SNS response, allowing the stressor to produce an adaptation of constructive growth and development. The key to training is to challenge the body repeatedly within the range of a constructive SNS response.

STAYING IN THE SWEET SPOT OF ACTIVATION

Training conditions the body to handle stress. What was once stressful becomes simple. There is power in therapeutically stressing our body. The power of adaptation works in tandem here as well. The purpose of the stress response is to adapt to the stressor. In training, the stress response of our body, as it is challenged, is managed by the SNS and driven by the emotion brain.

SNS/PNS ROLES IN TRAINING

The purpose of training is creating effective adaptation to increasing levels of challenge. This is crucial in training the autonomic nervous system as well. Assimilating stress, low grade stress, or put another way, therapeutic stress, causes the body to adapt and normalize the stress. When it does this, the body no longer registers the event as a stressful event. This changes the dynamic of the autonomic nervous input. The key with training the SNS/PNS system is to press the line of "emergency" stress to real emergencies and allow the body to engage in low grade emergency drill exercises to teach the body to no longer view those as emergency incidents. When this occurs, the flood of high stress hormones reduces and the body is able to engage a challenging activity without entering the extremes of SNS activation. These extremes are the freeze, flight or fight response of "emergency" stress. For an athlete, this is counterproductive. We need a sweet spot in autonomic training. When an athlete skips foundation training and attempts to train at a level too far beyond their current abilities, the body goes into emergency stress response and the training is undermined by the flood of stress hormones. It's important to train diligently and remain in a constructive zone for autonomic activation. This is often severely overtrained in the name of "no pain, no gain". The problem with this is that the gain is undermined. Undermining our training efforts is not adapting to the intelligent design of our bodies. Remember, working within our inherent design is what will unlock those more effortless expressions of strength and conditioning. Undermining training creates injuries, holes in the training foundation and is often a symptom of impatience in discipline. Discipline is building a solid foundation. Rash movements and advances attempt to build on a faulty foundation.

The PNS role in training is predominant in recovery. Taking the time to recover in our training regimen is the key to building our body to adapt to the stress of the training stimulus. The PNS stimulates digestion, allowing our nutrition intake to replenish the energy used and build the adaptation effects within our body.

PNS & DIGESTION, WHAT'S FOR DINNER?

The digestive system is important to peak performance. It details how the nutrients we eat enter our bodies and are broken down into smaller components that are able to be absorbed into our bodies through the lining of the digestive tract. Once these smaller components are absorbed in the body, a process we call assimilation, it is used as fuel and a builder of cellular regeneration. As a quick side note, our body attains its energy fuel through the air we breathe in, meaning atmospheric gases that help us drive our body's systems, as well as the food we eat. These are the two sources of energy for our bodies! Here, we'll focus on the digestive system, discussing the system's operations as well as the food we ingest and how that relates to the system and is used by our bodies.

MACRONUTRIENTS AND MICRONUTRIENTS

There are two categories to the nutrients we eat: macronutrients and micronutrients. The macronutrients we eat consist of a mixture of carbohydrates, proteins and fats. Included within the mixture is also the micronutrients, which are minerals, vitamins, enzymes and all the extras associated with our food sources. They include the organic compounds as well as the inorganic compounds that our body uses. This is important to know because these compounds are complex in our foods, yet, our digestive system breaks this complexity down to its most basic forms so that it can be assimilated into our bodies through the lining of the digestive tract. Then, these simple and basic substances go through a process of rebuilding into new structures through what we call biochemistry! If you don't think that is pretty amazing, I'm not sure if you are breathing! So, what is biochemistry? It is all the complex chemical reactions in our body that basically reorganize the components from our inhaled and ingested energy sources (food and the air we breathe) into usable forms of energy as well as the regeneration of our body's cells. Side note: Our bodies go through a process called mitosis. Weird word, I know. Basically, it is how our body recycles and regenerates itself. When cells age, they get recycled and our bodies go through a cycle of renewal on a regular basis. We are what we eat has some literal truth to it!

Now, organic compounds are the larger, more complex substances and the inorganic compounds are the less complex substances. Organic compounds have certain bonds in them called covalent bonds as well as certain elements called carbon - carbon and carbon - hydrogen. These two qualities of organic compounds makes them very difficult to reorganize in the biochemical processes of the body. Meaning, they are not easily separated and reorganized into something else. This is good because some things in our bodies need to remain stable. Now, inorganic compounds and substances are things like water, salts, acids and bases. They are substances that are held together by what we call ionic bonds and are easily broken to be used readily in biochemical reactions. Ionic bonds are electrostatic bonds and are what create an electric current in our bodies. We need electric currents to drive nerve impulses, use of electrolytes and various functions of the body. Both organic and inorganic substances are equally important to the body's function, survival and its ability to thrive. Both are a part of the food we ingest.

The food we ingest includes the macronutrients of carbohydrates (which are largely organic compounds due to the C-C bonds and C-H bonds present within them), proteins and fats. These macronutrients are one of our main energy sources for cellular metabolism and cellular respiration. Combined with the oxygen we breathe in, these help produce energy for our bodies to do work. Neatly, the energy demand dictates how these nutrients are used.

As we ingest our meals, with their mixture of carbohydrates, proteins and fats, our mouths begin to mechanically break down the complex structure of the food with the use of our teeth. In addition, the glands in our mouth secrete enzymes that chemically break down the bonds that hold the complex structure of food together. At the most basic level, all substances are made of atoms, which are then bound together through various chemical elements (such as carbon, hydrogen, peptides, etc) by chemical bonds. The bonds are broken in chemical reactions and enzymes catalyze those reactions, meaning they make them happen! As our teeth mechanically break down the food we ingest, the enzymes begin chemically breaking the bonds in the food. Now, the purpose of digestion is to take the complex structure of food and break it down into its most basic parts so that our bodies are able to re-assemble them into other structures or use them to drive other chemical reactions in the body, like energy production for athletic work.

ENERGY PRODUCES ATHLETIC WORK

Work could be a number of things such as running, walking, our cells reproducing and replenishing themselves, our organs becoming efficient in their purposes (such as the liver clearing our bodies from toxins more efficiently, muscles contracting, blood pumping, lungs expanding, and so on). Our bodies are always working even when we are resting and they need a steady supply of energy to do so. This is called the basal (resting) metabolism, meaning it is the most basic energy production needed for the body to maintain its factory operations and not close its doors for business. Work above that baseline requires more energy production as well as more energy input in the form of food and the air we breathe. The more energy output, the more energy input is required. This is why caloric intake must increase when more athletic demand is placed on the body. We can get into the types of energy input in a later section. The energy input is important. With an increase in demand in athletic work, an increase in energy intake is needed.

ENERGY OUT NEEDS ENERGY IN

As food is broken down in the mouth, it travels down the esophagus and enters the stomach. Here, it is combined with (HCL) acid and the turbulent mixing and churning of the stomach. In addition, the (pancreas and gall bladder) glands secrete further hormones into the mixture. Some of the components are absorbed through the lining of the stomach and into the blood stream at this point. Remaining components are released into the small intestine where the environment is not as acidic and further enzymes and hormones work to break down the food into its most basic forms. The most basic forms are as follows: for carbohydrates, it is glucose, sucrose, galactose, and fructose, starch and fiber; for proteins, amino acids; and for fats, glycerol, fatty acids and phosphate groups.

Food is assimilated at various points along the digestive tract as the enzymes released within it do the work of chemical break down. Transporting across the digestive tract lining, carbohydrate and protein derivatives enter the blood stream in the capillaries that surround the lining of the digestive tract. Fat derivatives are absorbed differently than protein and carbohydrate derivatives. The gall bladder releases a substance that creates what are called micelles. Micelles surround the fat components in the small intestine and then are absorbed into the lymphatic system surrounding the intestines. They circulate through the body's lymphatic circulation, re-entering the body's blood circulation at the major vein near the heart.

Food compounds, both organic and inorganic, get ingested at the start of the digestive system, which is our mouths, and then are progressively broken down as they travel to the remaining parts of our digestive system. What is not assimilated into the body is eliminated. What is taken in and stored for energy use is managed by the hormonal system. The hormonal system is influenced by interaction of our nervous system, the two faces of the champ within toggling to move the body into action or rest. When in rest, food is broken down, assimilated into the body and stored. When in action, food, in the form of stored energy, is mobilized and delivered where the internal action is happening.

ENERGY TRANSFER BEGINS DEEP

Energy within these organic and inorganic compounds, ingested from our food sources, is housed in the chemical bonds. As the interactive interplay of sporting relationship occurs outwardly, that interactive energy exchange runs deeper to that of the smallest parts of our bodies. Our cells. Producing athletic work through the exchange of energy. Energy releasing in the bonds of our stored food components to ignite movement and action. Flowing from the inside out, energy transfer creates interaction.

Chemical bonds are what allow our bodies to create electric charge as well as build and regenerate our body's structure and functional abilities throughout recovery. Compared to covalent bonding, ionic bonds are more easily released. They are dissolvable in blood and interstitial fluid, which is the internal sea our cells live within. Energy stored within these bonds is released into the body, becoming the kick behind the athletic energy released in the game. Harnessing energy from the food we eat centers on chemical reactions within the body. Hormones control when the energy is released and when it is stored. Hormones are directed by the two faces of the champ within. The autonomic nervous system impacts our hormonal system and directs energy in the form of catabolism or anabolism.

ENERGY TRANSFER - REARRANGING & RECYCLING

Energy transfer occurs because energy is conserved and recycled, it is not consumed. Chemical reactions rearrange energy to be expressed differently in our world. They are like a rearrangement and reorganization of substances. Put another way, they are like the rearranging of furniture in a home or a remodeling of the existing components to create something rather different. This is the art of energy transfer and recycling. Reusing energy allows life to be sustained, creating interactive and vital relationships. Energy is what brings actions to life. It is what moves us and it is how we are impacted and moved upon in this world. In sport, energy is the point of it all. Harnessing peak performance is living vibrantly, deeply engaging in the exchange of energy to bring greater expressions of athletic work to the game.

NUTRITION INTAKE DRIVES ENERGY TRANSFER
(FROM THE FOOD WE EAT ON THE PLATE TO THE SOCCER KICK, IT'S ALL RELATED...)

We have energy sources in the oxygen we breathe in as well as the food we ingest, digest and assimilate. This is important because energy is where we derive our ability to perform at our peak. To extend energy from the champ within, there must be energy available in stored nutrition.

Foods carry a nutritional profile that are a mix of carbohydrate, protein and fats. Whole food components are not solely one macronutrient. Unless, you're looking at straight sugar or straight butter for dinner. Not very tasty. Whole food sources have a predominant macronutrient profile. This is where we get diets that are described as high carbohydrate or high protein and the foods that accommodate the shift toward those predominant macronutrients. Foods like breads, pastas, vegetables, fruits and grains have a predominant carbohydrate nutritional profile, yet also carry protein and fat derivatives at a lower percentage of the whole. The proteins that we ingest are a complex mixture of amino acids in food form. There are essential amino acids and non-essential amino acids. The essential amino acids are those that we must ingest for our bodies to maintain optimal health and wellness; our bodies cannot make them. The non-essential amino acids are those that our bodies are able to produce and are not essential in our diets for our bodies to survive. The fats that we ingest are a complex form of fatty acids, omegas, and glycerol components. These sources of nutritional energy keep life and energy flowing in our body. Our body needs energy to survive and thrive.

Now that we understand these macronutrients in food form, let's dive into the way our bodies break them down and then use them in metabolism. Metabolism is the use of our nutrition and food in the energy production systems of our body, generally known as our bioenergetic systems. These systems are the ways our body replenishes internal energy stores from the nutrients we eat and the oxygen supply we breathe as we exert physical energy and use up those resources. Remember, energy out requires energy in. Rearranging and recycling. Energy flow. Energy transfer from the inside out and back again.

We discussed previously how the digestive system helps us enjoy these nutrients and then allows our bodies to absorb the sources of energy as the smallest units of their structures; that is the simple sugars, amino acids, fatty acids and glycerol. Once the broken down aspects of our food source is assimilated into our bodies, some of them are used immediately to fuel the work of our cellular processes. Remember, our cells are working around the clock to do the specific jobs they were designed to do as well as the process of mitosis. Mitosis is the constant regeneration and renewal of our cells in our body and requires energy to do so. Thus, again we are speaking about our basal metabolic energy demand. The energy we use to survive and exist.

THE ATHLETIC ENERGY SHIFT - SURVIVING TO THRIVING

While a baseline amount of the energy we take in is used for survival, the remaining stored energy becomes available to shift beyond the energy focus of survival. Taking a close look at the way our bodies harness and release energy tells us that the body is not made only to survive. There is more to the existence of such an incredible living organism than the mere survival of its basic mechanisms. Humans were made for more than existence. They were made for impact. Adaptation tells us that. We either rise or resign, develop or regress, according to what we do with energy transfer. Shifting from survival, the athletic work places a demand on the body that elevates its expression. Do you not stand in awe when excellence is expressed?

Development, growth and progression is the shift from surviving and maintaining. It is the launch of a thriving body. The impact of that energy expression touching and impacting our world around us. The expression, of which, elevates and transfers the energy into those around us. Have you ever been moved, impacted, motivated by the thriving energy output in someone close to you? Ever felt the "lift" of their presence? The very nature of thriving is lifting. Elevating. We are relational creatures. What happens around us influences us. It is good for humanity to elevate. It is good for thriving to populate and perpetuate among us. Energy is caught, it is transferred. It is transferred within us in the foods we eat, it is transferred and reverberated through us in the release of that energy out of our body. It is like a ripple effect, moving through us to those around us. Mobilizing them, energizing them and encouraging them. Emboldened and lifted, they begin to resonate and come into harmony with the energy of the lift. Athletic thriving is good for the soul. Athletic thriving is good for humanity because thriving lifts and elevates one another. To sabotage a thriving expression is to rob the world of constructive energy! Thrive! Shake off the dust of unbelief and fear. Champions were made to rise.

HARNESSING ENERGY IN OUR FOOD SOURCE TO THRIVE

Energy, from the base nutrients in our meal, once digested to a storable form, is stored in our bodies. Transferring energy from the food on our plate to the soccer kick on the field is the art of harnessing and releasing energy! The components of our macromolecules, carbohydrate, protein and fat, are sitting before us at our dinner table. Those components represent the energy while the body's design goes to work to transform that energy, recycle it and rearrange it. Once it's been recycled, rearranged and reorganized in the process of dismantling digestion and then chemical reactions, energy transfer ignites within and extends without. While we rest, we eat. When we eat, the first phase of that process is completed. Energy is stored as potential for work. Parasympathetic engagement. The face of rest and recovery. The resting champ is refueling. When we become active, the second phase of harnessing energy is completed. Energy is routed out of storage, sent to work and released through chemical reactions. The release is reverberated, resounding and impacting. From the inside out, the force of the energy within brings life and energy to our world.

The food sources in our macronutrients carry the energy for release. We carry that into our body when we sit down for meals with one another. The food on our plate. How does it work? The delectable combination that sweetens our taste buds has an ulterior motive! The enjoyment of food meets a deep need within. Of course, harnessing that enjoyment to serve that need is what peak performance is about. Discipline, but not without its enjoyment. We have taste buds for a reason!

How does our body work to transfer their energy? Internally, there are processes to convert all forms of macronutrients, carbohydrate, protein and fat, into energy. Ideally, each macronutrient has a particular thriving use within our body but our body has work-arounds within its production systems for survival, if needed, and its not afraid to use them! Intelligence. Intelligent design.

When pursuing the thriving expression of athletic work, combining the use of these nutrients to work for the peak performance is crucial. Shifting the body from surviving to thriving creates a solid foundation of stability for higher level work to launch from. To thrive, protein is best preserved and harnessed to build aspects of our bodies, while carbohydrates and fats are best preserved for energy production. The combination of carbohydrates to fats is crucial for energy. Too little carb intake and the body shifts into survival energy production and away from thriving and building. Too much fat intake and the body becomes thicker with less strength capacity, less agile mobility and more insulation than what is needed. That insulation infiltrates outwardly and inwardly. Stored as excess underneath our skin layers, stored around our organs and even within our arteries, the clogging feature of an overabundance of this nutrient ranges from presenting as an additional obstacle reducing effective movement to life endangering blockage of blood flow in the form of clogged arteries. Getting this ratio in the constructive and building zone is crucial for survival in its extreme as well as thriving when our energy needs extreme focus and development. Surviving is one thing, thriving is another. The body will survive over thrive if it ever has to choose between the two. It is best to not put the body in the position to demand a choice! In athletic development, this is absolutely crucial. Avoiding this predicament will avoid the undermining it creates in training efforts. Training smart. Intelligent training. Cleaning up the holes in the foundation starts with intact maintenance of survival. Robbing Peter to pay Paul destroys it all. The delicate balance of building is done on a foundation that is not indebted. Live abundantly. Honor the basics.

On a different note, fats are actually nutrient dense. Micronutrient dense. Vitamin and mineral dense. Within the macromolecule profile of our hamburger lies the smaller nutrients that are important as well. In the right proportions, fat intake serves our body well, so don't hate too much on the fat cells, ok. They are important too. On a cautionary note, they are also a place where the toxins we ingest are also stored. This is a good place to hate. And this is another good place to take to heart the phrase, "we are what we eat". Eat junk, store junk. Eat good, store good nutrients. Remember this when our bodies begin breaking down fat to produce energy. We want the nutrient dense fat as we are producing energy, not the toxins. *The nutrients released in fat metabolism will continue to nourish our efforts and build an efficient system. The toxins will burden our systems and create some issues and inefficiency in that effort.*

CARB LOADING

For healthy individuals, the source that is used first and primarily in exercise is glucose. It is the preferred source of nutrition for energy production. The next source is fat and then, only if needed, do we begin to use protein. It is ideal to avoid using protein as an energy derivative for athletic expression because protein is meant to build our bodies. *If we have exhausted all our energy sources stored within the body, and must revert to protein, we are basically breaking down our bodies to energize our bodies. This is counterproductive and undermines the purpose of work and peak performance training.* Protein supplementation and intake is absolutely crucial to athletic development. It plays a part in the recovery and building side of training, primarily when the face of the champ is switched to rest and the parasympathetic nervous system is gearing the body into adaptation. Training effect. The effect of training is built by protein. The energy to train is built best through carb and fat use. It's important to understand the primary role in these macromolecules and how they relate to the two sides of the champ as well as the two aspects of training. It will make or break the athletic pursuit of peak performance.

As an athlete, you've likely heard the term "carb loading". This is mainly done among endurance athletes and it is loading the body with carbohydrate energy. A high carbohydrate content meal, such as pasta, is eaten the evening before an endurance event. This excess carbohydrate is digested and then stored in the liver and muscle cells, becoming available when the body runs low on blood glucose. It is loaded energy. Designed to keep the body functioning in the carb/fat ratio of energy production, it protects the protein reserve needed during recovery.

Immediately, the energy in carbohydrates is used for survival work as the blood glucose elevates after a meal. The shift between the survival and thriving use of carb energy is controlled by the hormones. Once the survival needs are met, the excess carb energy is then converted to starch and glycogen to be stored in our liver and muscle cells for later retrieval when energy demands get high again.

When carb loading, excess energy is stored in preparation and expectation of making a very steep demand for energy thereafter. The ability to keep the body using carb/fat ratio stores during athletic work keeps the body in a thriving mode. When the carb and fat stores deplete or are inefficient to supply energy, the body begins to break down protein to supply it. In doing so, the foundation of stability that has been built is now being converted for our energy expenditure. Carb loading, especially in endurance athletic work, keeps the body from reaching in and undoing the work already laid in previous training sessions.

ENERGY OVERVIEW

Cellular metabolism is the process by which our body converts all of these macronutrients into glucose to produce adenosine triphosphate (ATP). ATP is the pure energy transfer. It is what is transferred from the food on our plate to the soccer kick in the game! The connecting point between energy in and energy out hinges on ATP. It hinges on unpacking it from our food and mobilizing it deeply within our body to fuel action, movement and productivity. From the potential energy being stored within the body to the kinetic energy being released in activity and production, the energy ingested is harnessed by the incredible intelligence of our internal mechanisms and released in productive work!

Once the active face of the champ is on, the sympathetic nervous system on fire, the hormones mobilize the food stored within, sending them to their destination. Chemical reactions occur that take what is available within us and create energy for the demand our body is under. While there are many workarounds and ways our body is able to compensate for energy production, harnessing the use of energy, both in nutrition intake and in conditioning of our energetic production, is necessary for the finely tuned athlete to hit their peak. The greater development attained, the greater the focused and efficient use of the energy production is required.

GAME FACE AND ENERGY INTERCHANGE

The game face of our champ has two sides. Recovery and resting, the champ builds potential. Energy is brought into the body. Energy within the body is used to build greater potential in the champ. Potential energy. Stored, developed. The power of parasympathetic nervous stimulation lays the champ to rest to build greater potential. Active engagement, ignited by the other side of the game face, the sympathetic system, takes that built potential and expresses it powerfully. Kinetic energy. Released. Impacting. This ebb and flow of energy in and energy out is the expression of sport interaction. Fine tuned over and over on the solid foundation of constructive growth, the athlete stands taller, climbs higher, reaches for greater peaks and rises again and again. The heart of a champion rises. How does the heart, the emotion brain, impact and drive energy exchange deep within the body all the way out to the interaction of sport? The emotion brain has the power to lift. Champions rise. Harnessing that power takes balance and precision. A balanced emotion brain ignites and empowers champions.

THE IMPORTANCE OF A BALANCED EMOTION BRAIN

While the emotion brain moves us, why is it important that it be a balanced and healthy movement? How does what motivates a person affect the SNS/PNS responses within our bodies? The emotion brain is the switch to the autonomic nervous system. It is also the barometer, so to speak. With the power to alter intensity, the emotion brain balances the two faces of the champ within. Harnessing energy, driving the body into peak performance, the emotion brain keeps the body steady and controlled to cross the finish line. Without this yin and yang balance of these two faces of the champ, what is left are the extremes of loss of control. The opposite of harnessing energy is energy gone chaotic or wild. Without self control. Without focus. The two faces of the champ become the gin and yank of an out of control crash and burn. Burn out. Overload. Tanked. Potential energy used and wasted. Potential lost. The expression of work crashed on the shore of energy gone bad. Sometimes, we use the word "toxic" or "destructive" to describe situations like that. Those two terms define what the use of energy looks like when it is not harnessed and focused. Instead of peak performance, what results is the opposite. Destruction. Break down. Development undone. Foundation destroyed. Not only is there a shift from thriving to survival thinking but now, the body shifts from survival to recovery. Recovering the "normal" maintenance foundation due to reckless and rash uses of energy. The gin and yank of an imbalanced emotion brain not only has the power to limit peak ability, it also, left unchecked, has the power to destroy normal survival maintenance within the body. It's really not worth neglecting. It's the driver of the athletic base. Imagine what gin does to the driver? Yanking them off the path and crashing them, it destroys constructive growth.

The harmony within a healthy emotion brain resonates like yin and yang, ebbing and flowing, creating rhythm and harmony. Resonating, developing, fine-tuning. Rising and soaring. Do you see the difference? Driving our body's actions can either be a smooth and progressive operator, yin-ing and yang-ing along the mountain edges like hind's feet, or an out of control drunk, gin-ing and yank-ing all over the paved road in front of them.

THE MAIN PLAYERS OF THE EMOTION BRAIN

Comprised of the limbic system, the emotion brain creates the tone of the body. That emotional tone ripples through the physical body with its effects via the autonomic system activation and engagement. Think about that for a moment. What ignites the champ within? What engages both the active and engaged champ and the resting/recovering champ? The autonomic nervous system! Kicking off input from the emotion brain, the SNS/PNS toggle the switch between the two and even determine the intensity of that activation hitting the nerve networks. Some of those networks travel along the spinal cord, others impact the hormonal system. Hormones create a cascade effect and either switch on rest, digest and recover with the PNS activation or activate the mobilization of energy stores for the engagement of action with the SNS activation. Hormones and nervous impulses travel through the body, preparing the face of the champ needed to step forward. The occasion calls and the champion arises. Ebbing and flowing in a harmonious ease of productivity outwardly and then inwardly. Over and over. Energy in and energy out. Building the champ within. The expression of the champ coming out in the impact in the game.

The players of the emotion brain are in the limbic system. They include the amygdala, epithalamus, thalamus and hypothalamus. Crazy names, right? Just thought I'd make some introductions. Each of them are congregated and connected right in the center and the heart of the brain. The amygdala is an extension of one of the basal ganglia components. The hypothalamus sits below the thalamus. Above the thalamus, the epithalamus sits closest to the amygdala. The seat of our motivations. Motivations are what moves us. What moves us impacts us in many ways and one of the major ways it impacts us is at the (hypothalamus-pituitary axis) HPA axis. The hypothalamus is a part of the HPA axis.

The HPA axis is a connection between the brain (nervous tissue) and hormones (endocrine system cascade). While the hypothalamus is an extension of our brain and its nervous tissue, the pituitary is a part of the hormone system. It is an endocrine gland and releases hormones into the bloodstream to flood the body. This HPA axis is the connector between these two systems. It is stimulated by influences from the amygdala. The amygdala is the emotional regulator of our emotion brain. When the autonomic nervous system is influenced in the amygdala, it impacts the hormones at the HPA axis. What does this mean? It means what motivates us determines the state of our body. Are we moved to action (sympathetic nervous input) or are we moved to rest (parasympathetic nervous input)? What moves you?

THE MOTIVES OF THE AMYGDALA

Deep within the heart of the brain, our emotions are felt, processed and acted upon. Much like the way we sense our environment in the literal, we sense emotions around us as well as respond emotionally in interaction. Unable to physically touch this aspect of our sensing ability, it is what some call a "sixth sense". It is catching the emotional sense, the cultural sense of a community, a person or a situation. The impact on our soul depends on the intensity of the emotional thrust around us. Unhealthy souls impose and leak out destructive emotions. Those are emotions of malice, ill will, jealousy, envy, gossip, arrogance, and I am sure the list goes on further to include other destructive type of emotional expressions. When a soul is exploding with those type of destructive emotions, like a live wire, it is felt everywhere. The toxic entanglement of a soul in those gutteral groans is a soul stuck. Following the brain, the body becomes stuck. Restricted. Unable to lift against the weight of an imbalanced emotion brain, the body hits its ceiling. The ceiling is the emotion brain. Lift the lid of destructive emotions and the entire tone of the body changes. That emotional tone drives home a response in the autonomic nervous system, cleaning out destructive energy and harnessing clean and pristine actions from the inside out. Obstacles removed, energy that is uplifting floods into the amygdala and the tide turns. At the HPA axis, the driver is smooth, coordinated and balanced. The yin and yang lays to rest the gin and yank of those destructive motives. What moves you? What moves you to act? Do you see the power of the motive? It sets the tone for the entire body.

THE HPA AXIS DRIVER - SMOOTH OPERATOR

The HPA axis is the meeting point between our brain and our hormonal control. It is interesting that the two main modes of communication within our body are the electrical conduction of our impressive nervous system and the cascade effect of our interactive hormonal system. Both of these communication modes prepare wide and varied organ functions that serve the same purpose.

When we think about systems integration, it requires complex movements and a synchronization of system operations. Even further, the synchronization is of only specific functions in the systems within the body, meaning the hormones and nervous impulse travel the body enter various organs and turn on extremely specific functions. Sophistication like this is driven at the HPA axis by the autonomic nervous system! The communication from the brain through its nervous system and hormonal system has a series of communications that prime the body for collective and specific action. Specificity of training. This is where sport specific training helps harness these very specific and complicated interactions. Specific training primes specifics in the body to serve a higher purpose, directed by the command and higher processing centers in the brain. The two faces of the champ, the active or resting champ, moving and turning on switches all over the body. Unrestrained and yet, globally specific in its operations. Building and waking the champ within. Powerful interplay.

Systems integration, in athletics, is predicated heavily on neuromuscular and hormonal fitness. Does this not make sense? Can you see the close connections between the brain, the autonomic nervous system and the hormone interactions? Neuromuscular control has deep and far-reaching effects. So does hormonal communication. Our nervous networks are electrical conduction pathways that span our entire body much like our blood vessel networks. Communication from the command center, our brain, flows through both. That begins at the HPA axis, in the center of the brain. The communication is an outflow within both the blood stream and electric nervous system. The body is switched on and directed.

The effect of the nervous system impacts the HPA. The limbic system, a main player in our emotion brain, influences what is stimulated in the HPA; whether that is parasympathetic activation/sympathetic inhibition or sympathetic activation/ parasympathetic inhibition. To rest and recover or to act and engage is influenced by our motivation. Remember that the emotion brain is the motivator. What moves you? Negative emotional constructs or more healthy emotional constructs?

The emotional overtone of our mind affects our hormones by responding through the nervous system input. Fear, anger, emotional pain, grief all have powerful effects on the body. Ever witness the power of fear dismantle a well trained athlete or a performer on stage caught in performance anxiety? It's real. Fear, felt and processed in the emotion brain, has the power to disable physical ability. Anger, left uncontrolled, creates destruction and real consequences in lives. Emotional pain causes a ripple effect in the body. It can cripple a body just as heavily as physical pain. Grief has the power to move a person to a new beginning, and yet, it also has the power to cause someone to be blocked and stuck in life. The power of emotions.

While much of these type of emotions create obstacles, negative effects and destructive outcomes, there are constructive ways to process through them. Everyone feels a wide range of emotion. We are emotional beings with a powerful emotion brain. Learning to harness it and allow it to work for peak performance is so much wiser than attempting to deny its existence or shut its voice off. It doesn't stop speaking. Not listening to it will cause its voice to be heard in other ways. Other more destructive and unhelpful ways. Propping up in disease process, elevated stress, hormone imbalance, dysregulated nervous system function, muscle tension, headaches, health issues, the emotion brain impacts and touches every part of our body one way or another. It cannot be denied because it is. Denying it is like pretending that your femur doesn't exist. How does that work? The point is is that it doesn't work. Right.

SNS HORMONE CASCADE IN THE CHALLENGE

The active and engaged autonomic nervous system, the sympathetic nervous system, activated the body through both the spinal cord and the hormonal system. At the HPA axis, the nervous impulse in the brain electrically lights up the part that releases a hormone cascade throughout the body. This cascade touches glands, causing them to release substances within the blood. The specific gland that functions strongly with the SNS is the adrenal gland. Sitting atop the kidneys, each gland is stimulated to release adrenaline and noradrenaline when the SNS is activated in the brain. These hormones, circulating wildly in the blood, create the "emergency" stress response. The internal 911 activation code, so to speak! As the hormones circulate, our body heightens to action and responds like an emergency responder. Body is on high alert and moving quickly. Adrenaline levels high. The intensity of the body's response is determined by the intensity of the sympathetic innervation at the HPA axis. What alerted that? The emotion brain. Sensing a threat, the amygdala swings into action and pulls the body into alignment with that action. In true emergencies, this is crucial.

Keeping the emotion brain balanced and healthy keeps the emergency responses preserved for those needs. It also keeps the intensity of the activation of the SNS and its hormone cascade appropriate to the level of stress. What is training? Training is stressing the body. Conditioning the emotion brain to handle the stress of training without kicking in an emergency level stress response is what keeps the athlete grounded in the game.

PNS HORMONE CASCADE IN THE RECOVERY

Recovery is the name of the game in PNS activation. Laying the champ to rest, the PNS shifts the tide and energy focus of the body. Switching off the hormonal control of retrieving stored energy and turning on the hormones that begin rebuilding, repairing, strengthening and adapting the body to the stress. With recovery, the body goes into rest, rehydrating and eating. The hormones shift into digestion and storing energy. It's a different ballgame. The yin and yang of the champ. Precept upon precept and line upon line, the champ is built with every new challenge. The heart of a champion rises, no matter how many challenges come. A champ stands up and faces the game. Built in the heat of the game, in the heat of energy transfer, in the heat of sport interaction.

MAINTAINING THE HEALTH OF THE TWO FACES WITHIN

While the heart of a champion rises, there are circumstances that can crush the health of a champ. Recall that the two faces toggling on and off in the expression of the champ are driven either harmoniously or recklessly. Yin and yang, or gin and yank at the wheel. That driver is the emotion brain. What does that mean? It means our motives matter. Healthy motives maintain healthy driving at the HPA axis. Healthy driving creates healthy flow of ANS stimulation and expression of both faces of the champ within. Healthy ANS stimulation and intensity keeps the body yin-ing and yang-ing, expressing athleticism in a pristine and clean development of excellence.

CHAPTER SIX

THE ENEMY OF PEAK PERFORMANCE HAS TWO FACES

Enemy. What a strong word. Aversive. The enemy of performing at peak is the antagonist present in your path of intelligent training. That antagonist being the dead weight dragging on an athlete, draining energy like water attempting to be held in a cracked jar. Energy meant to build, leaking out for what purpose? There is no purpose. There is no focus. There is no meaning to the enemy of peak performance. What is the enemy? It is the unharnessed use of energy, the energy waste. Like a maniac, destroying good things, tearing through constructive territory and ripping apart decent developments, unfocused energy leads to systems disintegration. Chaotic and dissonant, the enemy of peak performance destroys the foundation in an athlete and disrupts the forward momentum in training. With no sense, no rhyme or reason, it dismantles and destroys. Why go along with something so destructive to peak performance?

The opposite of performing at one's peak is the descent into dysfunction, disease and disability. Where there was potential for great ability, the energy drain disables that vision and writes a new one. That new vision is the opposite of peak performance. It is disability and disease, dysfunction and destructive constructs. Energy dismantled, systems disintegration and disorder leads to loss of energy. Loss of energy leads to ineffective and inefficient athletic work. Ineffective work leads to demotivation and despair. A loss of momentum breaks the spirit of an athlete. An athlete is bred to progress. It's wired in them. It's why they love the training. Breaking progress, sidelining momentum is breaking the heart of an athlete at their core. Dragging along unawares, the novice athlete stumbling down a path that will cost more than they understand. Naive. Unlearned. Unaware. Until now.

THE MISUSE OF ENERGY

Recall that sport interaction is the interaction of energy. That energy comes full circle. Ingested, food is broken down, assimilated and stored as small units. When needed, it is retrieved, unpacked. The energy is then transferred from the depth of the body to the bat, striking the baseball in a line drive projection, just shy of third base. Energy enters the body, goes deep, is transformed and harnessed and then explodes out of the body in athletic work! That is sport interaction.

Misusing energy is dismantling that full circle operation, adding obstacles within it, and slowing its transaction. Instead of heading toward a fine tuned presentation, the progression shifts toward the negative training effect. The receipt, the transfer and the expression is negatively affected away from the target vision. While there are many factors that lead to a misuse of energy, there are some that can be intelligently bypassed. Remember that training is a cause and effect relationship. While there are many things in life we cannot control, there are some things that we can. Choosing the cause of an effect is one of them. Meaning, there are two ways to train. Intelligently or foolishly. Wisely or ignorantly. With understanding or carelessly. If we go through a training regimen, do we not have the power to choose its path? Do we not have the power to create an intelligent path? We do. The misuse of energy in training occurs when the body is subjected to a training stimulus that is no longer in the sweet spot of an athlete's constructive challenge zone. In other words, the athlete is training either below or above that zone. Training above it is over-conditioning while training below it is under-conditioning.

HARNESSING ALIGNMENT

Harnessing energy and bringing it into alignment with a training target is the point of intelligent training. Alignment. Laying out a vision, assessing the point where one is at and where that vision is projected to take one, is the beginning of intelligent training. Bringing an athlete into alignment with that vision brings that vision to life in that athlete. Resonance. What is vision but a divine alignment? Excellent pursuits resonate. What one pursues is what is built within. From outward to inward and rebounding back outward in expression, the vision is casted, internalized, and released in athletic expression. Spending time developing the vision is time well spent. It is the defining target built and raised within the champ.

Training is the process of aligning the athlete and the vision until they are one and the same! Raising the vision before the eyes like a target one is aiming toward becomes the resonating development in the heart of an athlete. Helping and guiding an athlete along a path of intelligent training brings to life the peak expression of athletic expression within them. It is the athlete's desire to move toward the vision. Without that desire, there is no vision realization. No development. No internalization. Activating and releasing an athlete is like releasing arrows from a bow along a straight trajectory, straight into the heart of its bull's eye. Yet, alignment requires and commands respect for the desire to be aligned. Training is both casting vision and matching vision. Intelligent training is casting peak performance in an athlete that deeply desires the realization of that vision within them!

THE DICHOTOMY OF VISION

Where there are two visions, there is division. Casting a vision and creating alignment first begins with agreement. How can two walk together on a journey unless the finish line is the same line within them both? Destination is the point of a journey. The vision of the finish line is the point of the path. Aligning the visions, developing authentic agreement and building resonance at the onset of the race is just as important as the race. With its projected finish line, the start aligns the finish. Shooting out the gate, at the sound of the gun flaring and signaling the athletes forward, a course is set. Direction. Movement. That course leads, defines. It guides. It directs and maintains the path to the vision. Realizing vision starts as the athlete decides to step into the blocks, position their feet and prepare for the launch out of the gate. They know where they are headed. Desire within them is aligned as they align their body at the start of the journey.

Dichotomous visions are disharmonious. Pulling in two directions, whether within an athlete or between an athlete and a leader, it dismantles energy and focus. Dissonance, the opposite of resonance, begins. Undermining the path, working against the vision, this pulling in two directions pulls a person apart. Disintegration. While peak performance is predicated on systems integration, its opposite counter effect is realized with dichotomous vision and systems disintegration. The misuse of energy, unleashed and chaotically spinning out of control, takes a finely tuned potential in an athlete and crashes them in burn out and untapped potential.

Bringing alignment from the inside out, from the beginning to the finish, is building a unification toward one vision. Ownership of vision. Vision must be owned because it is the vision that shifts from an outward target to an inward development. The champ sees their target in front of them, yet, in crossing the finish line, looking within, they realize the target within them is what moved them over the finish line. They are the target, the race and journey the tools of development. They are the vision, the vision within of the developed champ, crossing the finish line. Alignment at the start, stepping into the race, progressing and building, becomes the alignment within as the champ crosses over. Culminating a finish, the reward rests in the hands of the champ. While representing outward attainment, it is the inward development that propelled them to the finish.

Dichotomy is the opposite of alignment. Dissonance is the opposite of resonance. Division is the opposite of vision. Disable is the opposite of able. Chaotic disorganization is the opposite of clean and pristine. Two paths, a fork in the road, the moment of decision is at hand. Choosing the path, aligning oneself with the vision, the choice is in the hand of the contender, the athlete. Choose. Choose well. Choose with the end in mind.

TRAINING IN BOUNDS

With the end in mind and the choice made, what is next? Resonating with the vision at the starting line is the beginning, but there's more. Activating desire and sparking connection to the vision, the sound of the gun signals the start of a race. With momentum and ignited motivation, the vision compels the athlete forward out of the gate and into the race. Stepping onto the rough terrain of challenges, the path to the end is riddled with tests, obstacles and intentional difficulties. Their presence has an aligning purpose. Testing the athlete, demanding the intelligent design to elevate within them, the challenge builds the champion in the crucible of training. There is rest for the weary. While the testing is intense, the recovery stations allow the champ to internalize the effect of the challenge. Cause and effect playing out as the athlete traverses the peaks and valleys of training.

Losing one's way in the journey is inevitable at times. Going before the athlete, the leader casts the vision over and over, keeping the direction before the eyes of the contender. It is the eye that directs attention, builds direction and maintains focus. Focus is the unifying force in building resonance. Building resonance is the purpose of the training journey. Placing the vision before the athlete keeps them in bounds and remaining on the path as the rough terrain of training presses their limits and challenges their focus.

THE SPARK AT THE TRAINING EDGE

Challenge is the point of the journey and it is this challenge that reveals the training edge in the athlete over and over. What is that training edge? It's the point where the challenge sparks the edge of the athlete's abilities. Like iron hitting iron, a spark ignites between the two. Building a passion for more, the body reaches for it, stretching to a new height. Going for it, expending the remaining energy within them, the effort exhausts the athlete to momentary depletion. Limit felt, body exhausted, energy spent, the currency of training begins to build a return as recovery develops, replenishes and grows the champ within. The training edge, exposed in the power of challenge, is covered in the quiet grace and involuntary process of internal recovery.

Power and grace. Challenge and rest. Effort and stillness. Depleted and filled. Explosive and built. Spent and earned. Expended and developed. The paradoxical and pointed training edge. Sparking. The fire of heat and energy exploding within as energy is transferred in the interaction of sport. Igniting life, growth, development at the edge of what is within, the heat builds. Cliff hanging in a figurative sense, the champ is built in the heat of the moment, burning bright at the training edge.

Trust. Trust is built at the edge, where the voluntary effort expressed outwardly meets the involuntary response developed inwardly. Trust the innate design. It is the intelligence housed within the body, quietly building and igniting an involuntary grace lift. Resting in the lift, the champ is built on the graceful mechanisms of the body's internal machinery. Working in the background, this involuntary and innate process is unfettered and unseen by the conscious awareness of the athlete. Trust. Trust the process. In rest and quietness, the inner strength emerges. In recovery, the body is built. Power and grace intertwine at the meeting place of an athlete's training edge, developing and building the champ.

HARNESSING THE SWEET SPOT AT THE TRAINING EDGE

Harnessing energy and aiming it to spark at the training edge is the point of intelligent training. It's the point where two unite, those two unifying pieces being the athlete's unique design and training limit and the intelligent understanding of the human body. The sweet spot of training for any athlete is highly individual. Remember that the athlete is a living organism, distinct and fingerprinted with a unique stamp that cannot be organically duplicated. Striking the match of their training edge is only done with intelligent and deep study of the athlete's unique characteristics and developments. What works to ignite development in one athlete doesn't necessarily work for another.

What unites the unique athlete and the intelligent development of their design? A leader, trainer, healthcare professional, sports coach, mentor, fellow athlete, you name it. Anyone that takes it upon themselves to invest intelligently in an athlete through an energetic and mutually enjoyable interchange is capable of serving in that role. Athletes love training and often choose mentors, coaches and the like to enlist help as they prepare to grow into the next level. The harnessing of that training edge is built by a village, surrounding and supporting the athlete as they step into the crucible of training and development. Investing in the development of an athlete is the heart of a leader. Leaders invest. As the reward of that investment rises to the occasion and looks them in the eye, the satisfaction of a finish line crossed runs deeper than the act. What is developed and harnessed within the athlete is the sweet spot for the leader.

Sparking the training edge and igniting the flame of transformation is best done in a therapeutic and building relationship between a leader and an athlete. Leading the very unique athletic characteristics of an athlete into the crucible and mixing the intelligent design of the human body, the leader and guide builds an encounter between the two. The power encounter. It's the power encounter that precedes the lift of grace. It's the voluntary effort preceding the involuntary response. This sweet spot, facilitated and focused by the leader, defines the bounds of intelligent training. It is the building ground of growth and development. Missing the mark, even slightly in one direction or another, causes the trajectory of the arrow to fly off target. The realization of peak performance requires consistent focus and perseverance to train within that sweet spot. An intelligent harnessing of transformation at the training edge, igniting explosive power, is tethered by the strength of the athlete's leaders, guides and most treasured influencers.

TRAINING OUT OF BOUNDS, MISSING THE MARK

Development undone, unwound, unharnessed and unfocused leads to chaos and disorder. The opposite of developing peak performance, unharnessed energy twists the process of focus into chaos. While there are varying levels of expression in a lack of focus, it is unfortunate to see peak potential and opportunity unwind and flatline. Did you ever notice how the excitement builds when an athlete is about to peak and explode past the finish line? The crowd anticipating the victory and instinctively roaring for it! Is it not inherent in the heart of humanity to desire peak development? Is it not the glory revealed in the human body to display its excellence, igniting and lifting a movement among us as it does so? Ingrained deep within is the desire to witness growth, development and progress in the fine-tuned and pristine athlete! It's human nature to develop and grow.

Training out of bounds begins when the spark is missed. Without the spark and power of the training edge, there is no transformation, no real growth and no development. There may be incredible effort and a grand display of busy work, but unless the training edge is found and harnessed toward the vision, the sweet spot is lost and the effort ineffective. Ineffective in the realization of an inward desire. Ineffective in the internalization of the vision. Missing the mark one is aiming for, training out of bounds, is the loss of the sweet spot, the loss of focus, the loss of vision.

Developing the sweet spot is the work of leading. Self discipline is an athlete's ability to lead one's self toward a projected finish line. Developing relationships with chosen mentors allows others to bring experience and expertise into that development process. Fine-tuning the training stimulus to match the training edge in the athlete is the spark that keeps the vision alive. It's a concerted effort to maintain. Between the athlete and the mentors they choose, the pitfalls of training can be avoided.

THE TWO FACED ENEMY REVEALED

On either side of the path and journey are pitfalls. Pitfalls in the training and pitfalls in the athlete. As we traverse the focused journey, weed through the obstacles, and discern the excellent from the wasteful pursuits, our vision for the path becomes sharpened. With the help of intelligent mentors, pitfalls are exposed and dismantled. What are these pitfalls? They are the internal and external moments of opportunity to miss the mark, miss the spark.

Externally, the major pitfalls of intelligent training fall within the training parameters. It is the overshooting and undershooting of the training stimulus, commonly called over-conditioning and under-conditioning. These two training errors become the two faced enemy of an athlete's development. Engaging in a training stimulus that over extends the training spark in an athlete leads to breakdown. This overextension takes on many forms. From a training stimulus that presses far past the peak training zone, the therapeutic building zone, the sweet spot of development to a training recovery that gives the body no opportunity to maximize off the training effort, no time to allow the involuntary and automatic process of internal development. *While over-conditioning creates an over-stimulated athlete, under-conditioning creates a de-conditioned athlete.* Engaging in a training stimulus that is not strong enough to engage the spark of the training edge never allows the edge to be felt, challenged. Playing it safe, under-conditioning becomes a self limiting and ineffective effort. This under extension can take many forms as well. From inconsistent training, too little effort exerted, lack of accountability to great effort but too much time spent in recovery, thus losing the momentum of athletic progression.

Internally, the major pitfalls of intelligent training fall within the training limits of the athlete. Specifically, they fall within the ways the athlete perceives their training limits. Having a growth mindset is crucial to athletic development. Expecting the results of the finish line before the finish line is attained will drive an athlete into despair and demotivation quick. Despair and demotivation breaks momentum and progress.

Champions are built in the process. Development, when standing at the finish line, looks different than the development when shooting out the gate at the start. Training edges are developed in the process. The line of that training edge, moving forward regularly as the training effect lifts the athlete from the inside out in recovery. The development in the journey, making room for the developments of the champ. With each step through the race and journey of development, that edge progresses until the athlete accomplishes the vision, crossing the finish line, built from the battle and crucible of the journey.

Maintaining a growth mindset, understanding that the process is a process, limits the damaging effects of an unhealthy emotion brain and its destructive constructs. Keeping the mind out of perfectionistic, all or nothing, fail or die, splitting and condemning ways of thinking about one's own progress helps take one off the chopping block of hostility and place themselves in the crucible of enjoyable growth and development. Growth is not only a destination, it is a process. Making room for that process, especially when one is in it, creates the peaceful emotional resonance that fuels motivation and perseverance. Keeping both alive and strong is what gets an athlete over the finish. Crushing the spirit are the harsh and demanding self talk, condemning and critical in nature and desirous of tearing down rather than building a champ. A champ is built, not torn. Keeping the mind resonating in emotional intelligence and health keeps the body progressing, developing and growing toward the finish line.

THE GIN AND YANK OF A DYSREGULATED NERVOUS SYSTEM

While the very real penalties for conditioning out of bounds leads to over-conditioning or under-conditioning, the effect of that misapplied training hits straight into the nervous system. Training effects are real. There are effects to training even when the training misses the mark. A dysregulated nervous system is one of those effects. There are many other effects, but this one has a far reaching effect on the body because the nervous system reaches deep into the body of an athlete.

Recall that the two faces of a champ center around the toggle switch functioning of the autonomic nervous system. The yin and yang, harmonious expression of the champ is two sided. The sympathetic expression is the active and engaged champ, voluntary in movement and conscious in effort. The parasympathetic expression is the recovering and restful champ, involuntary in internal development and mostly unconscious in that effort. In health, these systems ebb and flow with the training regimen. Creating a training effect that keeps them balanced while progressing an athlete forward is the key to intelligent training. It is also the key to keeping these systems working for the vision of peak performance. Unfortunately, the potential for great focus and peak ability leaves open the potential for its opposite effect. When the training misses the mark, creates a negative training effect, that effect hits square into these two faces of the champ.

We are influenced by our environment and our environment is influenced by us. We see this play out between the cause and effect of training. With the training stimulus, our bodies are influenced to adapt and grow. In a negative training stimulus, one that misses the mark, there is an effect. A negative effect.

To recap, the two faces of the champ within mirror the two aspects of the training without. What does this mean for the autonomic nervous system? It means not only does the healthy functioning autonomic nervous system impact the ability to engage in challenge but the challenge has the ability to influence the autonomic nervous system functioning. Pulling the functioning ANS out of balance is striking a dissonant chord somewhere in this two step interaction. Either the training effect drove the ANS function down into dysregulation or the the dysregulated ANS drove the training down. Do you see the downward spiral of dysfunction? Dysfunction takes a champ down. It disables and dismantles healthy functioning. Moving from the harmonious yin and yang of peak performance progression, the dysregulation drives performance into a downward spiral of chaotic destruction. The dissonant chord building momentum within the body, developing ground and winding the nervous system into greater levels of chaos and disorder. The effects of which span all aspects of the body that the autonomic nervous system touches and interacts with. We know, by now, that those are far and wide throughout the body. From the heart, lungs, brain, blood vessels, emotions, intellect and beyond, the reverberating effects of a downward spiraling champ is a defeated champ. Like an out of control driver, the emotion brain spirals out of control and crashes the vision.

A dysregulated autonomic nervous system starts with a small misplaced training effect. Cumulative, over time, the training projection and effect shift off course and so does the nervous system as it adapts to the new direction. Unless there is a shift back on course, the training guides the nervous system, driving it into dysregulation. We are influenced by our environment, what we experience, what we take in, what we subject ourselves to. That is why the training has an effect on our body! Peak performance works to harness that training effort to build a champion that resonates with power and development.

The good news is that we also influence our environment. Overcoming a challenge is what champions do. We are impacted but we also impact and overcome. Coming back to the place where the pitfalls of training affect us internally, recall that our attitudes, thoughts and motives also drive us. While a training effect has the power to impact our brain and dysregulate our autonomic nervous system, our brain has the power to impact right back! The power of focus in thoughts and attitudes. The power of healthy emotional constructs. The power of driving the driver from the command center and overcoming the training effect is in itself an adaptation in emotional strength and mental fortitude. Stay in the game, it's not over.

What does the driver drive? The two faces of the champ within, the expression of which is regulated by the two sides of the autonomic nervous system. What does it mean to drive the driver from the command center? The driver of our autonomic nervous system, one of its main influencers is the emotion brain.

Emotional energy, healthy emotional constructs and attitudes have the power to elevate the body when the environment is attempting to tank its system out of balance. Gin and tank may have taken the wheel in training, but yin and yang still have the wheel at the command center, if we so choose. Bringing balance back into the nervous system is affected either through a training stimulus or the power of the emotion brain. We influence our environment and our environment influences us.

The limbic system of the emotion brain drives the ANS response from the command center, but the influence goes in both directions. The training stimulus activates the SNS and impacts the limbic system. In the training stimulus, we impact and are impacted. That impact is felt deeply and responds deeply.

Overstimulated SNS, under-stimulated PNS. These two toggling aspects of the autonomic system work in tandem. When one is heavily stimulated, the other is heavily inhibited. A training effect engages the SNS because this is the side of the champ that moves and acts! More commonly, it is the SNS that becomes overstimulated and creates dysregulation because the movement in our body is voluntary and movement impacts the SNS all the way to the emotion brain. Positively and negatively, there is opportunity for impact. Positively, it lifts the mood. Ever felt down, discouraged and stuck and decided to get a work out in just to have that mood lifted? How about training so much without rest and recovery that your body hits a wall, affecting your ability to think clearly, producing mental and physical fatigue? The SNS drives and turns the body on for activity through processes that are not under our direct control. Those processes are automatic and involuntary. Yet the act of movement is a voluntary act and creates an indirect impact on the SNS!

THE GIN OF OVER-CONDITIONING

Over-conditioning is a process of putting the SNS on overdrive and flooding our bloodstream with stress hormones that press beyond the constructive training zone and begin creating strong undermining cracks underneath us. With cracks developing in the foundation of the training, the body has slipped into a self-sabotaging dysfunction.

The yin and yang becomes the gin and yank. The excess stimulation drives the SNS into an anxious state of activity. There is no longer a sense of stillness in the effort. Have you ever seen an athlete all wound up and amped up? What is on the inside reverberates outward and you feel it even though it cannot be touched or looked at directly. It starts to unsettle you. Like a frenzied rumble, unable to relax, the stress from within driving the productivity of that athlete like a harsh taskmaster, perpetuating fear upon fear. Recklessness is the expression of the soul as you look in the eye. The nonverbal expressing insecurity and tainting every action with its unsettling grip.

Have you ever seen an athlete steadily engaging in intense physical work with a deep settled peace in their eyes and nonverbal expressions. It almost seems like a striking paradox. We often think that more is more, where obviously, in cases like this, less is more. Put another way, energy harnessed and expressed in a focused manner, removing the extra effort of psychological stress while enduring a physically stressful activity.

The difference between these two athletes is in the balance of the autonomic nervous system. One is highly dysregulated, hyper-active and on overdrive. The energy pumping through the emotion brain and exerting effort like water leaking out of a jar. The other is highly regulated, active and alert, yet psychologically still. The response of the autonomic nervous system is not misplaced into an extreme expression. It serves the purpose of peak performance.

Staying in bounds creates a harmony and interplay in our body but stepping out of bounds in either direction leads to disharmony. Systems integration is our goal, remember. When we move out of bounds, we begin to develop system disintegration and pull apart at the seems. Like a ship with bolts missing, a crash and burn is in the very near future. This is evident in the regulation of our autonomic nervous functioning as well as our emotion brain. Both of which are tied and influence one another.

THE YANK OF UNDER-CONDITIONING

Adaptation works in both directions. Under-conditioning occurs when our training does not challenge the body enough to create a shift in adaptation toward peak performance and the goals within our sport. Instead, it either remains at maintenance or sadly, it regresses the line and one becomes de-conditioned. There is a fine line between finely tuned, conditioned athlete and the process of de-conditioning. The key to peak performance is to find that line in an athlete and cause it to shift in the direction of an intentional goal with a training stimulus.

The point at which an athlete begins to undo the hard work of development is the beginning of a resigned champ. As our adaptation response shifts into the negative, de-conditioning begins to set in. When the line has regressed beyond maintenance and into de-conditioning, issues of disease have opportunity to crop in. While many individuals can be powerfully conditioned in the face of disease, others develop diseases because of the risk factors that occur with de-conditioning. There are a whole host of illnesses that develop due to the break down in our physical activity. De-conditioning not only creates a negative training effect, it can also lead us into an extreme negative effect of disease and disability.

De-conditioning shifts the balance between the PNS/SNS toward predominant and overactive PNS activation. PNS activation is important for digestion, protein synthesis, body building mechanisms. It's the place that adaptation builds or depletes. The body will adapt to the demand placed on it. Without a demand, it progressively weakens. Either the body is steadily downgraded and becomes weak or it is steadily upgraded and becomes increasingly conditioned. With under-conditioning, the body weakens.

When the PNS is overstimulated, the body is not conditioned to act when it needs to act. This would be the difference between decisively dropping into the center of a wave versus remaining on the board waiting for wave after wave after wave to pass. It is checking out, floating and disengaging into a chill zone when the time to act and engage is now.

Think about it like this. There is a line that you stand at. It is your current abilities. Toeing that line everyday and challenging it will press the bounds forward. Retreating from that line, will shift it further back on you as you step back. If the retreating becomes a way of life, the body moves into a steady decline and sadly, even progressive illness and disease if it continues without a change in direction. This is the opposing side of peak performance. Systems are disintegrating and the resigned champ is choosing to undo themselves. This is the place of self-sabotage.

THE TETHERING SOURCE OF YIN AND YANG

Yin and yang is symbolic of the harmonious nervous system, keeping our body appropriately active, engaged and in a state of grounded confidence. To avoid sabotaging the training effort and driving our body into a state of stress and dysfunction, the tethering source of the emotion brain is crucial. The autonomic nervous system not only activates the body for action or rest, it also develops and perpetuates actions based on the emotional tone of the body. That emotional tone dials up or dials down the intensity of the active engagement. It also is the dial operator that switches the emergency response system on when the body needs to respond with high levels of adrenaline.

While the out of control actions of the autonomic nervous system perpetuates its effects throughout the body, the emotion brain has the power to harness that effect and bring it into a healthier expression. Turn the page and let's dive further into that!

CHAPTER SEVEN

HARNESSING THE POWER OF THE EMOTION BRAIN

Have you ever looked closely at the eyes of a champion engaged in their game? Sometimes, it's like the flame is real, the soul coming to life in their nonverbal expressions. The eyes tell you the state of the soul. The presence of a person tells you much about their inner world. Catching it more than grasping, it slips past your intellect, slips past your mind and moves straight to your heart. Before you realize it, you are moved by it. Impacted. It is the unspoken dignity, the inner champ emerging. There is a soul to a champ. A true nobility that surfaces when the heart is fully integrated and the passion is ignited. It's one of the reasons we stand in awe of them and watch them. It's one of the few aspects of a champion undiscussed, but deeply revered. We know when we are in the presence of a champion before they say a word and make a move. It is unnerving, uncanny and yet absolutely incredible. Commanding respect quietly, it draws that very quality out from the onlookers. A rare presence. Excellent. Great. Admirable. The heart of a champion. Fully alive. Let's take a closer look at what brings a champ to life.

Slipping beyond the eye, the nonverbal expressions on the face and the emotional tone of the body, what lies beneath that is the powerful emotion brain. Coloring all of our actions, words and interactions with an emotional feel and an unseen presence. It's a challenge to capture the soul's influence and describe it well. Trying to touch it doesn't work. Studying its expressions under the microscope is a challenge. Yet, there's no denying that it's there. Influencing, coloring, adding life to interactions. The fire behind the effort of athletic work, being one such expression. A powerful one at that, When it's on, it is on. Igniting a movement, building momentum, swaying a crowd, gathering focus inwardly and outwardly, its effect is real. Yet unseen in so many ways. We feel it, catch it. Coloring our world in much the same way that music adds context and meaning to our life. Harnessing the emotion brain, bringing its energy into the vision of growth, development and peak performance.

HOW THE EMOTION BRAIN IGNITES PERFORMANCE

Bringing life to performance, the emotion brain sets a soul alive with motivation, drive and perseverance in the face of challenges and difficulties. The defining overture of a champion is one who is backed up against a rock and a hard place and somehow is still able to come through the finish! It is the roar of that inner giant, standing up in an overcoming strength that astounds those watching, taking on the obstacles that most would resign and withdraw from. What is that roar within? What is the fiery flame of persistence that presses an athlete beyond the aches and pains, the stretch and strain, the challenges in the race? It is the heart of our brain. The emotion brain functions as much of what our world refers to as our heart.

Lying in the center of our brain, the emotion brain is located right above our brainstem. Being the heart of the brain, it is the tone of our body's expression. The nonverbal communication of our interaction. The power of the soul fully alive and vibrant in our actions. Ever meet someone whose tone was unsettling? Ever been that someone? We all have. The words "we can be right and wrong in how we apply that rightness" ring true, don't they? We can be right in the logistics of our actions and wrong in the emotional tone and intent of those same actions. In other words, while our cognitive brain has the right answer, our emotion brain delivered it in an unhealthy and less constructive manner.

SETTING THE TONE

While the emotion brain sets the tone in our body, it is the place culture is created. What is culture? It is our feel. It is how people experience us relationally. It is the meaning we associate to the activities in our lives. It is the good vibe versus the bad vibe sense. It is what some call negativity and others call inspiring. Ever been around a person that caused you to feel uplifted in their presence? Someone who believed in you even in your unbelief? Someone who looked at you and knew there was more, that you were made for more? Someone that saw your potential and called it out of you?

On the flip side, ever been around a person that only saw what you weren't? Only saw a severely negative outcome for you? So driven by their negative assessment, so committed to its realization, that they spoke it and spoke it until you became small in their eyes. Belittling behavior is dangerous because it squashes potential and destroys seeds of greatness within people. It sends the message of "be little!" when, lying dormant within us, is a potential, a giant within, a greatness, a champ, waiting to emerge. We weren't designed to be little or belittle one another. We were designed to lift, strengthen, and build one another. Dormant, within the very design of our body, is the inherent and natural movement toward growth and development. Calling that out, harnessing that and normalizing greatness is the hallmark of a healthy and vibrant, alive emotion brain!

It is the fine tuning and resonate emotion brain that is able to take our bodies out of the gutter of negativity, failure and toxic dump and shift it into empowering growth and possibility. It is the resonating emotion brain that destroys fear of failure and ignites passionate and constructive explosion toward destiny and greatness. This ability to see the possibility and believe in one's ability to get there is the motivating cord in an athlete's training regimen. It is what keeps the athlete showing up and making steady effort to engage the challenge of training.

THE BREATH OF LIFE TO OUR EFFORTS

The emotion brain breathes life into our efforts. It is the place belief of overcoming and victory keeps us in the training regimen. It is the consistent engagement of our lifelong effort, allowing the results of that regular training to speak for itself on the showcase of competition. The athlete is made in the crucible of training. What keeps an athlete showing up to that crucible is the motivating thread of a healthy emotion brain.

An unhealthy emotion brain will tank a person's potential. It will cause the defeated champ to sit on the bench, resigning and succumbing to a disheartened sadness. Did you ever notice that resignation is never a happy moment? Did you ever notice how bad and sad it feels to let go of your potential? Did you ever feel the power of depression in this area? The power of not overcoming, with wave after wave blowing over you, taking you under the heavy force of defeat? If you have lived long enough, you have tasted the bitterness of that pill. It's a cruel taskmaster and it won't relent.

Yet, conversely, I've met some athletes that have been like flowers blooming in concrete. Surrounding them are naysayers, hateful and unsupportive comments. The culture of unbelief. The culture declaring failure and negatively spewing words to tear down and destroy a person's potential. When the waves blow over you like this, one begins to understand the power of limbic lock. The weight of the negative culture creating power and overwhelming you. These athletes though. I've seen them miraculously stand anyway. Something inside them stood up. It is the rising of a dormant champ that cannot be contained. It may have been plummeted with the unhealthy limbic lock of the community surrounding them, but like a flower growing in concrete, it emerged. There is a special type of mental toughness that accompanies these champions. They have learned the art of personal belief that is not dependent on what surrounds them. It is a belief running from deep conviction. It is the power of the leader within them emerging. The power of the emotion brain leading in a new way. It is the breaking of ground. The concrete giving way to the new growth. It is the new thing. The power of that emergence shifting the tide and leading the emotional climate in a new direction. The contrast so clear, so bright.

DEVELOPING EMOTIONAL RESILIENCE

Much of what we do is dependent on how it makes us feel. The crucible of training flips that around. What we do becomes the driver of our emotional response. Without this turnaround, an athlete would never finish a race, remain consistent in training or develop the emotional resilience to tolerate the discomforts associated with physical exertion. Training the emotion brain to delight in the work rather than only work when it is delightful helps train the mind in an athlete.

The act of training is an athlete willingly subjecting themselves to progressive and consistent challenges. Challenges are not comfortable. Baseline emotional resilience helps an athlete press past the initial discomfort and tap into the inner resources within the emotion brain. Those inner resources become the undercurrents to the physical exertion at the point of exhaustion. It is in that moment, the point of exhaustion, that the emotion brain stirs that inner giant, roaring against the cry of discomfort within, to finish the race, cross the finish line and secure the victory. The lift of the emotion brain comes through when the physical body is depleted and ready to give in. Losing motivation. Losing steam. Energy tanking. At the last leg of the race, when it all seems over and the athlete really wonders if the finish is attainable, it is the emotion brain that engages the body to soar over the pain, over the discomfort, over the negative self talk and drive the finish home.

Training the emotional resilience of our brain is developing a healthy perspective on challenges. It is hardening the physical body as well as the psychological body of our soul to the discomforts of difficulties. Mental fortitude, emotional resilience is the ability to stay the course no matter how you feel, what is said around you, who is treating you well, who is or is not supporting you. Remaining steadfast toward a worthy goal of growth and development in the face of obstacles relationally, obstacles in self perception and thought. The finely tuned athlete does not look to what is around them to develop them. They develop the internal machinery and substance of greatness in the crucible of training, the spark at the training edge, the fire of transformation. Emotional resilience is developing an internal growth and barometer mindset. One that internalizes your emotional state being determined less with what happens around and more with what happens within you. Developing, growing and allowing that involuntary work of our gracious recovery mechanisms to build the champ within, the focus of the champ is on the work that only they are able to control: themselves. Becoming a person of substance is where significance is magnified. Weighty and impactful, a champ ignites hope, uplifts spirits and minds, creates belief and possibility and stirs the champ within others to rise.

THE RELATIONAL POWER OF LIMBIC LOCK

The power of the emotion brain reverberates beyond the athlete, impacting and stirring the crowd around them. When an athlete excitedly takes the ball into the end zone, he's not processing that moment in a state of depression or sadness. His nonverbal, emotional expressions are on fire! Body exploding with excitement, slamming through with a roar that ignites the entire crowd to their feet! That is the power of limbic lock. The roar within the champ, erupting from the emotion brain through the athlete's physical expression, coloring his every action with an emotional tone of palpable victory. Pressing though the crowd, the explosion of emotion travels like a shock wave, felt. Hearts moved, emotions taken on a journey with the champ. Resounding for days, spinning for hours, the victory told and retold to anyone that will listen. The power of limbic lock.

Limbic lock is the rhythmic attunement of an influential and deeply emotional moment. It is the impact of the soul. The individual resounding with the deepest guttural explosion of energy, deep within the emotion brain, influences the crowd. When an athlete is moving in resonance, in great precision and focus, in excellence of skill and heart, that explosive energy emerges and ripples through those around them.

The limbic lock of sporting interactions is everywhere! It's one of the greatest parts of watching sports. Watching the athlete prepare, train, enter the challenge and subject themselves to the difficulty of the journey and discipline, the investment returning in the pristine expression of clean athleticism moves the heart deeply. Entering in to the emotional space, rooting for the athlete, believing in them, the explosion across the finish line takes on a meaning that resonates deep. Deep down, sports touches the human need and drive to overcome! To step up to the plate and face the challenge has a noble theme that stirs the heart of humanity. The noble theme of growth and development, becoming a person of substance, building the champ within. Humanity is designed to develop. Limbic lock elevates humanity with the champ, stirring the emotional state and giving them a taste of how good it is to be built in the crucible of training! Inspiring, igniting, moving. The emotion brain moves a crowd through the power of limbic lock.

THE NOBLE MOTIVATIONS OF A CHAMP

Decisions to act, move and engage our energy kick off in our thinking, cognitive brain. The kick behind that decision is the motive. Motives are the work of the emotion brain. Cognitive processing is driven by the motive, derived and expressed from within the emotion brain. What moves us? The finely tuned athlete is moved by clean and healthy motives.

Healthy motivations are a product of good will. Healthy emotional constructs keep an athlete resonating with noble plans and purposes, Confidence, belief, sound judgment, grounded perspectives keeps the head of an athlete in line with the vision of peak performance. Healthy motives maintain focus on constructive pursuits and uses of energy. Remember that the athlete only has control over themselves and their training regimen. The champ is built within. The work of development is not outward, on others. It is inward, on personal development and the real work of progress and discipline. With this view in mind, the focus of an athlete stays steadily on what they have the power to change and impact. That focus is empowered by strong and healthy motives.

TRANSFORMATION IN MOTIVATIONS

In contrast, the motives that bring the emotion brain into a dissonant and destructive outlook are often stuck in self-defeat, self-doubt, condemnation, hypercritical judgments, perfectionistic demands, envious comparison and jealous striving. Sabotaging an athlete's focus, these motives move the body away from the focus of peak performance. Energy is expended in pursuit of actions that do not build the champ within and develop growth. Instead, they often lead the focus into areas that are not in the control of the athlete. For instance, the loss of focus could be in striving for acceptance among peers when the very nature of having peers is acceptance into a peer group, spending an inordinate amount of time obsessing over the neighbor's new car as they live their fabulous life unaware of your attention on them, uninvited meddling in the business of others, gossiping and comparing. The common thread in these actions is that the focus is on externals, the situations that an athlete has no real control over. When an athlete is training and developing, that development focus is on the substance within them. It is on developing the fortitude and strength to face the challenge in their game. The unhealthy emotional motivations are a distraction to personal development as well as to the relational strength of healthy bonding.

An athlete develops and trains to bring their impact to the game. That impact is built within them, not around them. An athlete's mindset is a mindset of lifting. Their motivation is to lift their abilities, not tear down the abilities around them to win. There is no development, no training required in that. It is what is within an athlete that causes them to soar above the challenge. Focusing on externals to win is like an athlete watering down a challenge to overcome it. That's not the point of the challenge. The challenge is meant to impact and develop the athlete. It doesn't change, the athlete does. Development. Progression. It's an inside work. Harnessing the mindset that embraces the gift of challenge is the key to transforming unhealthy motives into more productive and peak performing motivations. Building a champ requires a lift. Why would an athlete not want to be lifted to something more?

When the formative years of development bring an onslaught of unhealthy relational entanglements, with words coming from very meaningful connections forming the basis of our self constructs, our awareness of who we are to and in this world, is it any wonder why some athletes struggle fiercely with an internal obstacle? A psychological obstacle. What is the emotion brain but that which is the seat of how we view ourselves, how we believe the world views us and how we view the world around us? Is it not the proverbial filter that we take in our world's input and express ourselves to the world?

Wounds that run invisible and deep, affecting every interaction of our lives, including the interactions with our own abilities, perpetuate until we stop and notice their impact. Stopping, there is an opportunity to recognize the patterns and rewrite the story. The layers of unhealthy insinuations, unhelpful comments and misguided words can be closed at the gate of acceptance. The first step is to create a checkpoint. Notice what is driving the behavior and ask, "is that what I want to drive my behavior?". The driver will lead our actions. If it is unhealthy or even of an ill will, we can be sure that it will result in an unhealthy outcome. Clean and pristine athletics stems from clean motives. One cannot reach the heights of their abilities while nursing their emotion brain in the dumps of toxic thinking. The beauty of all this is that it can be cleaned. It's a situation that is not permanent.

Peak performance training will bring this all to the surface. Remember, it's only an obstacle, not a wall. Training is designed to remove obstacles and chaos in an athlete's abilities. It is designed to harness efficiency and maximize a complete integration between all involved systems. And the system that runs its root extensions into every other is the emotion brain. While the wave lifts under us in preparation for our debut, it is up to us to lift our emotion brain to a psychological height that unleashes the true potential of our body. The impact is real. To ignore this is a deep betrayal and self-sabotage. Setting every system up for success means attending to every system, every aspect of what drives you, ignites you and moves you. We have an emotional brain. It's true.

Self-destructive beliefs and thoughts create actions. Think about the times you were motivated to act because of a hurtful interaction. When you were slighted, did you accept that the person is a separate person and does not have the power to define your perceptions of yourself? Or did you absorb it without a checkpoint and capitulate to its ruthless demands, recklessly reacting? How many times have your training sessions become a revenge against a person's words spoken in hate and spite over your life? Words sting. And, if the relationship is deep, those words sting more. Words will come. Hateful, even spiteful comments will come. So will powerful, encouraging words. So will constructive and helpful words. So will words that strengthen and ignite you. The power is in you: which words are you going to allow to motivate you? Which words are you going to allow to move you? Words have power. But, only the power you give them. Choose your influential voices well. Choose your self talk well. Confidence is what causes an athlete to step into the game and it is what carries them over the finish line. A healthy emotion brain matters to peak performance.

Motives for training matter. It matters because it taps into the emotion brain, the driver of cognitive processing. The cognitive processor then drives the rest of the body. Clean motives keep the expression and fruit of training clean, pristine. Remember the vision of peak performance? The vision of clean and pristine athleticism. It starts here. It starts at the "why" of our actions. It starts at the motive. Why do you train? Is it to lift and elevate your abilities and create constructive impact in our world? It is that very motive that lifts you. Ironic, isn't it?

FOUNDATIONAL CRACKS CAN BE FILLED

Our view of ourselves is largely defined by our parents as we come into our formative years. There is tremendous power in the words and steering power of a parent. Their words can be, while imperfect, healthy. They can be the platform and solid foundation that we launch our impact off of. Unfortunately, words can also serve to undermine an athlete's foundation. You see, the words spoken over a forming brain, especially the emotion brain, build deep associations and patterns that become more automatic in adult life. None of us come out with perfect formative years. Yet, some athletes come out with varying levels of foundational holes in this arena.

The good news is that it truly takes a village to raise a person in their young years. There are many parents in a person's life. Anyone that steps in to mentor, invest and help grow a person simulates a parental role. The need was meant to be filled by biological parents, yet, the human heart transcends biology when needed and seems to match itself to those that provide the input to develop and grow. The power of community often fills in the gaps.

Training will expose those foundational issues. Sometimes this can be unsettling. The emotion brain exposes its foundation in a more experiential manner. When an athlete is pressing their abilities to the edge, the issues expose themselves. That is normal. That is good. It shows the obstacle that needs clearing. So, clear it. The first step is identifying it. The second step is identifying the solution. The third step is applying the solution. The fourth step is basking in the glory of a removed obstacle and a clearer path.

Just as much that our soul brings our bodies to life when it is vibrant and healthy, it also creates a stale physical expression when it is traumatized and wounded. Dealing with the foundational cracks mends the soul and allows the emotion brain to soar, lifting the athlete in the game.

MAINTAINING EMOTION BRAIN HEALTH IN TRAINING

The driver behind our motion goes beyond the intellect. It is the heart, the place we feel, the emotion brain. Our emotion brain is the seat our emotions are processed. What we feel matters. It carries inherent meaning and attaches that to the event those emotions stirred. Our experiences carry an emotional weight and memory with them. Within the emotion brain, the impact of our memories set a foundation for us to stand on. Training in a way that preserves the health of the emotion brain keeps it working for peak performance and resonating in systems integration.

Traumatic insults aimed psychologically at a soul when training is like building a house and kicking down its foundation at the same time. Preparing an athlete to reach their peak by disabling their emotion brain takes the passion and emotional power out of their athletic expression. It is creating a soulless athlete. One cannot insult and hold back the soul and wonder why the athlete is not realizing their potential. Have you ever looked into the eyes of an abused child? The telltale sign is the resignation in their eyes. It's a dead and beaten soul. The life and vivacious joy is stamped out. What's left is a shell of a body with no heart. Or, no healthy and functioning emotion brain.

The emotion brain is the passion behind the athlete. It is what fires them up, gets them to the starting line, sustains them in the stretch, and powers them over the finish line. The emotion brain impacts our hormonal state. Our hormonal state impacts our autonomic functioning. It's that same autonomic functioning that brings the athlete out in each of us. The emotion brain has the power to depress the mind and depressed minds are demotivated. Demotivated individuals don't rise to meet challenges. They resign and quit in the game. To say that the emotion brain is not involved in athletics is to cripple the driving force in it all.

So what makes the emotion brain healthy? If it is so interconnected and has the power to drive both our central processes and peripheral processes either on the heights of our potential or into the gutter of defeat, how does one harness the power of the emotion brain to work for peak performance? It seems the missing link, keeping the tone lighthearted and upbeat within our body and mind. An uplifted body is a body that lifts. Think about that. A heavy and defeated body is a body that is stuck in a rut.

Champions emerge on the heights. They continue to get up and face the challenge. Instead of drawing back, they step in. What drives them to stay present? When looking at the mountains in front of them, what causes them to keep climbing? When the finish line is not in view and the dirt is in their face, what drives them to continue?

There is a power in intrinsic motivation. It is being motivated from within. The emotion brain is a powerful motivator. It is also a powerful demotivator. The challenge of training is not in momentary effort. The challenge is in consistent engagement. It's the moments when no one is looking, the choice to retreat has no consequence other than the inner awareness that one betrayed their own desire. And, then a downward spiral begins if one continues to retreat.

Intrinsic motivation. The emotional strength to press past the internal and external negative constructs. Intrinsic negative constructs are self-doubt, insecurity, fear of failure, fear of exposure, the harsh critic, the badness of shame and self-loathing. Internal negative constructs are the destructive ways we process how we view ourselves. The truth-telling with the tone of these negative constructs is not helpful, but rather becomes mean, degrading, disrespectful and discouraging. Do you know what it means to discourage? It means to lose courage. Think about that. What is courage but the strength to face the challenge! Facing truth with healthy internal constructs is the sweet spot of emotion brain power. It is the unleashing of athletic potential.

THE LIFT OF TRAINING IS IN FACING TRUTH

Facing truth. What is training but the consistent challenge to expose weaknesses in order to develop them? Training is humbling. It takes courage to train. It takes courage to expose areas that need improvement. With a healthy construct and tone coursing through our emotion brain, that correcting and training produces constructive change. Instead of tearing down, it lifts as it points out weakness. It lifts because the purpose of the exposure is to strengthen, not to crush. Crushing an athlete's potential through crushing their spirit disables their inherent abilities absolutely.

What are external constructs? Limbic lock displays the power of influence in our community. Have you ever seen the power of negative emotions in a group setting? Have you ever seen hysteria and panic move an entire group to chaotic actions that are uncharacteristic of the individuals in them? This is the power of limbic lock. Remember that our limbic system is the part of our brain that creates emotional intelligence, relational skills and community skills. It defines the tone of our relational expression. When that tone is unhealthy and negative, it begins to weigh on the individuals surrounding it. Depending on the level of relational bond we have with an individual stuck in unhealthy constructs, our limbic system begins to feel the impact of theirs. We are relational creatures. We affect one another and we are impacted by one another, even in our emotion brain. More is caught than taught here. Limbic lock is when a group becomes locked into someone's emotional construct and the power of influence shifts their emotion brain into alignment with theirs. This has the power for great good, but it also has the power for great harm.

In peak performance training, harnessing the external constructs of the emotion brain includes choosing coaches, trainers and associates that keep your limbic system resonating in an uplifted manner. The external constructs are the influences we surround ourselves with and they are the voices that speak into the vulnerable places of exposure in training. Choose voices that respect the emotion brain and its power to release or resign the champ within.

CHAPTER EIGHT

PRACTICAL TIPS TO ATTUNE INTO YOUR PEAK PERFORMANCE

T he tips and take-aways from all that has been shared so far are compiled in this chapter. Speaking in metaphorical, emotion inspiring, vision casting, allegorical and instructional language, the practical applications are sometimes difficult to grasp. This section has some straightforward in-struction and insights that will help drive home some of the main concepts discussed. As an athlete, there is tremendous trust you are placing in the influencers you choose to surround yourself with. The trust you extend to those individuals is a gift. Your vulnerability in the process of development and willing-ness to put yourself in the crucible of training, courageously fac-ing the fire of transformation is admirable. May these tips fine tune the message, lift you in your endeavor and offer real insight into your training needs!

TIP #1: HEALTHY SNS TRAINING

A healthy SNS training effect is one that lifts and elevates you without driving your emotion brain into the gutter of toxic thinking. Remember, your SNS switches on the active champ in you. It is the face of your effort as you train in the challenge. Keeping it healthy is keeping your finger on the pulse of your stress. Stress ramping up in the challenge is a signal to you. In-stead of backing off the challenge, pay attention to what is hap-pening in your emotional tone and thoughts. Evaluate your thinking and ask yourself what is stressing you out. Wait and listen. Honor that signal, pay attention to it. Make room and make changes if needed as insights develop after listening to the emotion in the stress.

Protect your emotional energy. In all the areas of your life, you are impacted by the emotions of others as well as your own. We often bypass this because we don't see its impact like we see a handshake or a car driving by. When in an intense training season, where the focus is pointed and the stakes are high, pull back from overextending your emotional capacity. Where interactions or situations are steering your focus off course, put a pause on some of those, if possible, and make some space in your heart to focus on the task in front of you. Remember, your emotional energy is the driver of your SNS response and your SNS is the switch that powers the active champ in you. You don't want that SNS in overdrive due to high stress. It needs to be steady and balanced. Keep your emotional energy free to focus on the training and your sporting event.

Paying attention to the health of the emotion brain is keeping the yin and yang in the driver seat of your SNS operation. Remember, your SNS is your champ activator. You need it to drive with focused, harnessed energy. Avoiding the gin and yank of a neglected emotion brain in the driver seat will keep you from a crash and burn in your peak performance efforts. It's not worth it. Pay attention, notice and make adjustments to improve health in this area.

TIP # 2: NUTRITION AND PNS RECOVERY

Your PNS is the system that goes into high gear when your body is internalizing the effect of your training challenge. It is an involuntary process and you have no conscious control over it directly. Indirectly, it can be hampered by not allowing your body the physical rest and recovery that it needs to allow the energy to harness in to its processes. Because it's not something that is directly impacted by being active, it's easy to mis-place space for this in your training. It can seem odd to rest when you are aiming for a goal. It seems counterproductive to our thought process. I get that. Make space for it though. This is where your inner champ is being built by the intelligent and quiet design of your body. Making room for this process in your training regimen will maximize your training efforts. The saying "train smart, not hard" comes from this phenomenon. A short-cut here is like making great money and losing the paycheck. Cash in on your investment and effort and let the return develop within you.

Nutrition is key. Protein builds the body as it does its recovery work. A post workout meal/snack is crucial to keeping the energy replenishing in you as well as keeping your body from pulling energy from unwanted stored resources. Or, worse, tearing down your own body to recover its energy reserve and do the internal work of adapting to the challenge. Operating on a nutritional deficit undermines the building process and dismantles your training foundation. Pay attention to your nutrition to keep recovery working for you.

TIP #3: STAYING IN YOUR LANE, FOCUS

Your body is designed with a unique fingerprint. There is no other you out there. The diverse genetic pool is not organically duplicatable, which means you are predisposed to certain talents that are natural and inherent to your genetic design.

This is where the phrase, "what are you destined for?" comes from. Destiny is really a word that describes destination. In reality, what that phrase is really asking is "how are you going to impact the world with your unique design?". Destiny is where you are going. It's your destination in life. Because of your unique design, you have the ability to express an aspect of humanity that carries a measure of absolute uniqueness in it. That's really neat. In all our similarities, there is a fingerprinted expression that no one else can claim. Identity. We are deeply similar and yet distinct.

In athletics, there are distinctions in your design as well. Find those, own your lane. If performing at peak is your goal, harness that design within you and stay in that lane. If you are built to be a power athlete, be a power athlete. If you are designed for endurance work and you enjoy it, stay there. If you have a wide athletic base and cross over into more than one athletic profile, harness into that power. The point is you are designed for a specific purpose. Part of tapping into that design is intelligently understanding your body and working within its natural talents to maximize your unique potential.

TIP #4: CHANGE YOUR LANE, CHALLENGE

On the contrary, expand your horizons some and develop your capacity to do what is challenging to you. Staying in your lane is important to remain authentic and true to your design but that does not mean neglecting your body's general ability to develop your athletic parameters. Stay in your lane but don't be afraid to expand it! You were designed to grow and expand. In fact, that is the entire point of athletic training and conditioning. Limiting yourself and closing yourself off in a box is not the heart of an athlete. Expand, grow. Start in your lane, that is your sweet spot and develop from there! Enjoy the lift. Take us on the journey with you. When you lift, we lift. It's inspiring absolutely.

Well rounded athletes, while stronger in their natural talents, expand and change the parameters of their lane and become a well rounded yet focused athlete. A wide training foundation and a deep and high training focus is your goal. Your training foundation is your platform of stability. Reducing injuries and developing increasing levels of systems integration for all types of mobility, challenging your lane expands your lane. Expanding your lane is growth. Grow. That's the point of training.

TIP #5: CROSS TRAINING

Cross training is where you will best challenge your lane. Filling in training gaps in the foundation of your athletic base happens in cross training seasons. The wider your base, the stronger your launch. Developing athletic foundation is a progressive interplay between building wide in cross training and then building deep in sport specific training to launch high in peak performance. The width serves the depth and the height.

Imagine an inverted pyramid for a moment. Attempting to place a peak performing demand, a heavy weight, on a pointed and narrow foundation is like being top heavy and toggling on a pointed edge. There's no stability there. Healthy cross training flips that pyramid back on its base, allowing the deep focus and heavy lifting of sport specific training to soar high.

Progressive athletic pursuit stretches and presses the bounds of your body. Your body is meant to develop and grow. It's wise to stretch those horizons. While the cross training seasons are less focused on the sports you love, they serve that development well, keeping injuries to a minimum and building real substance in your body's ability to stand in your sport.

TIP #6: SPECIFICITY OF TRAINING

Alternating cross training with sport specific training over and over is what builds progressive athletic development within you. Sport specific training is just that. Specific. Movements in sport are often complex, integrated and involving an exciting and interesting mix of your body's systems. Developing the specific movement patterns of your sport builds motor memory and stores those memories for later use in your sport. Moving from a constant and very deliberate, painstakingly conscious effort of thought in training into an automatic, almost effortless movement pattern in the game is the power of building motor memory. You want that. Your mind is heavily engaged when you are in real time, game time. Whatever you can do to condition its need for less conscious focus and effort, the more that energy can be harnessed for the cognitive and emotion brain to process your real time interaction in the sport. Your brain needs head space in the game. You need real presence for the interaction of sport. You need to be present with your head in the game. Sport specific training that builds motor memory gives it that space.

TIP #7: MEDICAL EVALUATION CLEARANCE

As we have seen, there are definitely some complex and varied moving pieces to building your athletic skill. Athletic skill development is highly complex and integrated. With many parts involved, unity and a central purpose brings those parts into focus and cooperation. Remember, that is what systems integration is. In everyday living, that central purpose is to survive and maintain life, at all levels from cellular to whole body function. In pursuing further development, such as with peak performance, it is to go beyond that and thrive, given the right inputs and tools to do so. And thriving is what this book is about. Thriving is the pursuit of peak performance. Thriving is the developed expression of a mature athlete. You were designed to thrive!

Just as important as cross training is to sport specific training for athletic stability, healthy function and basic survival in the body is the stable base our efforts stand on to thrive. Laying the groundwork for your body to function in a healthy manner is the deepest base in building athletic foundation. If your body is not functioning well at baseline, any attempt to thrive will be undermined. Building on a faulty foundation doesn't work. Health is the first layer of your athleticism.

It is important to get a medical evaluation and be certain your body is not in a diseased state. If there is a diseased state operating and gaining foothold, it will hinder peak performance. Remember, peak performance and disease are on opposite ends of the spectrum of body functioning. Pursuing peak performance is moving away from disease, dysfunction, disorder and all the ways our body turns order and organization into chaos, wreaking havoc on its ability to perform. It is shifting from surviving to thriving.

Getting medically evaluated and having expert eyes on the most basic functioning of your body keeps your head in the game, keeps your body in the game. While cross training builds the base for deeper focus in sport specific training, medical evaluation builds the base for sport engagement. Sports medicine physicians as well as other medical and healthcare specialties are a key part in your peak performance team. They keep you in the game, in the training. Without this piece, everything built on the foundation of athletic development crumbles. Staying in the game requires a consistent attending to the base. Holes there have a deeper impact than anywhere else. The point is, you don't want holes at the base and, if you find some, deal quickly and decisively with them! Engage your medical and healthcare team and stay in your game.

TIP #8: NUTRITION & METABOLIC TRAINING

Nutrition is important in the context of metabolic demands. Specific to sport, metabolic training requires nutrients to sustain energy production. Part of the metabolic engine is the retrieval of stored energy from the food you ingest. The macromolecules of which include carbohydrates, proteins and fats. Derivatives of these macromolecules are stored within the body and retrieved when the metabolic engine is ignited in athleticism. The demand of the sport and the your current conditioning level is what switches on specific gears in that engine. Those gears include two fast energy producing systems and a slower energy producing system. All run simultaneously at times but shift according to nutrient supply in the form of stored food derivatives and availability of oxygen breathed in and circulating throughout the body in our blood stream, flooding into cells. The engine for metabolism is housed within every cell. What does this mean? It means that the cells (most active in athletic work) are where the body shunts blood. That blood carries the oxygen from your breath and the stored nutrients retrieved in the process. It is the combination or the lack of both, that drive the metabolic engine gears into specific energy producing systems.

Athletes that require fast and high amounts of energy run predominantly on the anaerobic metabolic gear and fatigue out quickly. The quick and high force development exceeds the speed with which oxygen is able to arrive and supply the metabolic engine of the cells. Gears shift. Energy produced without oxygen is done so at a high cost. The cost of fatigue onset. Lactic acid threshold. Body unable to keep up with its clearance rate, lactic acid builds and the athlete hits the proverbial wall of muscle fatigue. Cooked. Done. It's over. At least for now.

Athletes that require a steady and moderate to minimal amount of energy over a long period of time run predominantly on the aerobic metabolic gear. They fatigue less. Oxygen flowing through the blood and into the cells is in good supply, keeping the engine well oiled, so to speak. The athlete is sustained over the long haul while the body clears out metabolic waste easily and readily, keeping pace with production. There is no back up in the system, no impending wall tanking the energy production.

Wherever you land on the metabolic profiling in your sport, nutrition is important because much of what you ingest is stored for this very process. The macromolecules are one crucial piece that fuel athleticism via the engine of metabolism. The key players in energy expression being carbs and fats. The key player in building adaptation in response to the training being proteins. Proportions matter. Getting this correct will feed your metabolic engine and shift its gears to predominantly function in the areas that match your sport as well as build your body in recovery. It is crucial to harness the energy of the food you eat into the metabolic demand of your sport. Pay attention to your proportions.

TIP #9: PROPER EVALUATION OF YOUR SPORT

Sport analysis is often underestimated. Just as much as the comprehensive assessment of your physical abilities is needed, the comprehensive assessment of your sporting dynamics are needed as well. Intelligent training learns the context of the training. That context includes both the athlete and the sport, you and your game. Remember that sport is the interaction between an athlete and the game. It is you and your game. It is energy rebounding between the two. Studying the context of that rebound, how energy is transferred within it, and the ways movement expresses itself upon it, prepares your training program to match the context.

Evaluating a sport includes taking a deeper look at the game. Is it a solo athlete sporting event? Track and field events, cross country running, downhill skiing and snowboarding, competitive surfing, athletic swimming, diving competitions, body building events, and the many more excellent solo athletic endeavors worth mentioning are all inclusive of a sporting medium that functions between the athlete and the surface of the sport. Some include equipment that provides the catalyst for that interaction. The study of the surface as well as the equipment used to interact with that surface is wise. Is it a team athlete sporting event? Softball, football, soccer, basketball, hockey? What are the dynamics of the team? What are the specific roles and distinct characteristics of each team member?

There is another element in team sport that is different than solo sport. The leadership and cooperation of a team requires a team blending skill. Cohesive and constructive resonance builds, not only within the athlete and within the athlete's specific interaction in the game, but also within the team. The added element of resonance within the roles of team members takes resonance one step further in the game of sport. Building resonance within an athlete, within the athlete's relationship to the game and then further, within the team's expression of the integrated resonance of its team members. Greater resonance, greater impact. The key is leadership and steering the energy toward the purpose and mission of the team. Disintegrated focus dismantles a team and creates just as much potential in a negative direction as it was meant to create in a positive direction. That positive direction being peak performance and the negative direction, in its extreme, being disease and illness. The peak performing athlete moves freely with ease in their sport while the disintegrated athlete moves less freely with disease in their life. The key is to emphasize resonance and de-emphasize dissonance at every level of athletic training.

Not only is there different sporting dynamics, whether solo or team, there is also different surfaces to consider when analyzing the sport context. Developing deep understanding of your sport context helps match your training to your sport.

TIP # 10: MATCHING YOUR TRAINING TO YOUR SPORT

Coupled with the understanding of the foundations of health and fitness stability through medical care and cross training, the specific training your body needs in sport specific training lends to building another layer. Layer upon layer, the athlete is built. That next layer of development is the connection between you and your sporting surface and context.

Fine-tuning and developing the complexity of athletic ability requires not only that the foundations be set well, it also requires the layers being laid and built upon those foundations be set well. There is an order to building a complex organization. Developing peak athletic skill is complex. The greater the complexity, the greater need for organization. The greater the number of moving parts, the greater skill development needed to keep them functioning together. Fine-tuning is necessary to match training efforts into your sporting context.

As you grow in and through the layers of athletic organization, it's helpful to be aware that more of your energy will need to be focused and harnessed as you do so. Fine-tuning your sport engagement also fine-tunes the energy focus. Like the point of a rocket, the sharp edge of your athletic breakthrough explodes off of the foundation of the stable base laid in your training. Precept upon precept, line upon line, the building moves from general and broad to finely pointed and deeply focused. Harness and protect your energy as you move into seasons of focus.

TIP #11: SYSTEMS INTEGRATION TRAINING

There's another layer in the complex building of a champion. It is the integration of systems within you responding to the complexities in the sport specific training surrounding you. What is outwardly expressed through you is an excellent expression of what is inwardly happening within you. Full circle. It's happening. Layering, rising, layering, rising. Reaching at one level, rising to the next level. Line upon line. Building, one step at a time. Rising and resonating, developing and fine-tuning in the fire of transformation. Soon to be launching like a rocket, moved and empowered by the blazing fire beneath, elevating to the heights of peak performance. Engines are on, systems firing with communication, connection and readiness. Waiting for the command.

Similar to preparing the rocket to launch, the body systems within you are smoothing out their kinks, working out the obstacles and becoming more efficient as you train. As your training develops and challenges you into the greater width of broad cross training and the deeper height of sport specific training, that same level of complexity and organization builds in you. No longer working solely on one part of your athletic ability, the integration of your movements, mobilization of your energy and the explosion of your force production is released as your systems integrate. Releasing the impact of your athletic presence is releasing the compounding effect of every system adding its weight to the game of your sport! This is resonance.

Coming together, integrating. Waiting for the explosive decision and motivating signal of the emotion brain, your systems are primed and ready for launch.

TIP #12: SPORT INTEGRATION TRAINING

The crucible of training builds the champ in its fire of transformation, sparked at the training edge. Preparing to engage your game, the training has developed you. It's time to step into the context of your game and train "game smart". Sport specific training not only elevates the finer, more focused demands the sport places on the body, it brings the body into a deeper context of the sport. Evaluating the sporting context is crucial to bringing the athlete into a training spark that matches that context. Another layer of resonance built again, here, is at sport integration. As the evaluation leads the design of the sport specific training, its effect challenges you, integrating the details of that evaluation and another level of your training focus is developed. Be encouraged, you're almost there!

TIP #13: ATHLETE-SPORT INTEGRATION TRAINING

Finally, the launch is here. The crucible of training has built the champ from within. In the fire of transformation, preparations have been made. At the training edge, the spark of a champ igniting. Here we are. Systems, electrically lit up by the power of the nervous system, communicating, integrating, organizing and mobilizing the body into action. Heat building, the fire of your training edge burning beneath. Eyes focused, prepared and ready. The challenges that grappled you, tested you, attempted to dismantle you, became the tools for your preparation. A divine twist. Instead of tearing you down, the roar of the champ within you turned the tables on those challenges. Remember, the champ does not retreat. Stepping to the plate, putting it all on the line, bringing the strength of your athletic presence, your impact is prepared and waiting for engagement.

Signaling the start, the fire ignites beneath you. The power of your emotion brain firing explosive energy through your body. The roar builds, the guttural cry beginning its release from the depth of your soul. Momentum building, energy building, exploding forward, the champ launches from the base. Like a rocket, the lift of development empowers the launch into the height of peak performance! Lifted, launched, elevated. There you are, flowing with ease in your game, finely tuned. In mastering the game, the game elevated you. Harnessed. Developed. Focused. Well done.

The vision of peak performance. Casted at the beginning, the pristine and finely tuned athlete is the realization of the finish line. The sport, being the stage to reveal the incredible substance built in you, simply providing the opportunity to see you soar. Do you realize that you are the award? Standing on the podium, receiving your accolades, do you realize the greatest accolade is what is built within you? The substance of your development, it's worth the journey.

Resonance. What does it mean to resonate? An athlete aligning deeply with their sport is an example of resonance. It is two separate pieces to an interaction brought together, creating incredible harmony. For the athlete, it's what we see when the skill of the athlete matches the demand of the sport. Integrating, coming together in a manner that builds one on another, an athlete and their sport showcases the champ within like no other.

CHAPTER NINE

THE EMERGENCE OF
THE CHAMP WITHIN

Systems Integration. Clean and Pristine Athleticism. Emerging from the victory, the champ standing beyond the finish line, a surreal moment passing. Did that just happen? Emotions on a high, body still electric from it all. That inner roar slowly settling in. Its effect still resounding within. Reverberating, Ringing. Moment by moment, screenplays running through the mind. Processing. Taking it all in. Slowly calming. Nervous system unwinding from the explosive power, getting its bearings. Sitting in the moment. Basking in the victory. Winding down. Coming down from the mountain. Wild fire. It's a wild fire. Wild and yet, controlled, harnessed, fine-tuned. The paradox.

The fire of the champ within. Burning bright. The training edge striking that match. Now, a way of life. Recognizing the edge. Living in the transformation. There's no other way to live. Fully alive, the champ whispers, "I am the fire".

Peak performance. Constructive. Building. Healthy training. A training that does not undermine an athlete's efforts but, instead, builds over and over, layer upon layer and foundation upon foundation until the heights have been attained, bounding effortlessly over one mountain peak and another. Is it possible? Few go there. Is it really because few have dared? Or is it that many have dared but few have harnessed their intrinsic, intelligent design that unlocks their ability to truly soar? Here we are again. That missing link in our training. The champ disheartened, emotion brain unattended. Odd. What was often missed and dismissed is actually a key driver in it all.

The power of the emotion brain. Connecting both the central and peripheral parts of our body, it's influence extends to every part of the body. How does the emotion brain influence other areas in our body? It does so by systems integration. Bringing all the parts into alignment, motivating and moving them with a centered emotional culture, even in the flame of intensity. A healthy emotion brain keeps an athlete's head in the game as the fire is raging all around them. Unfettered. Unde-terred. Experiencing all the intensity of emotion and yet, steady.

What is peak performance other than a highly developed system? What is systems integration? It is a highly developed group of systems! What is integration? It is the smooth coordination of those systems, operating under the peace of the emotion brain.

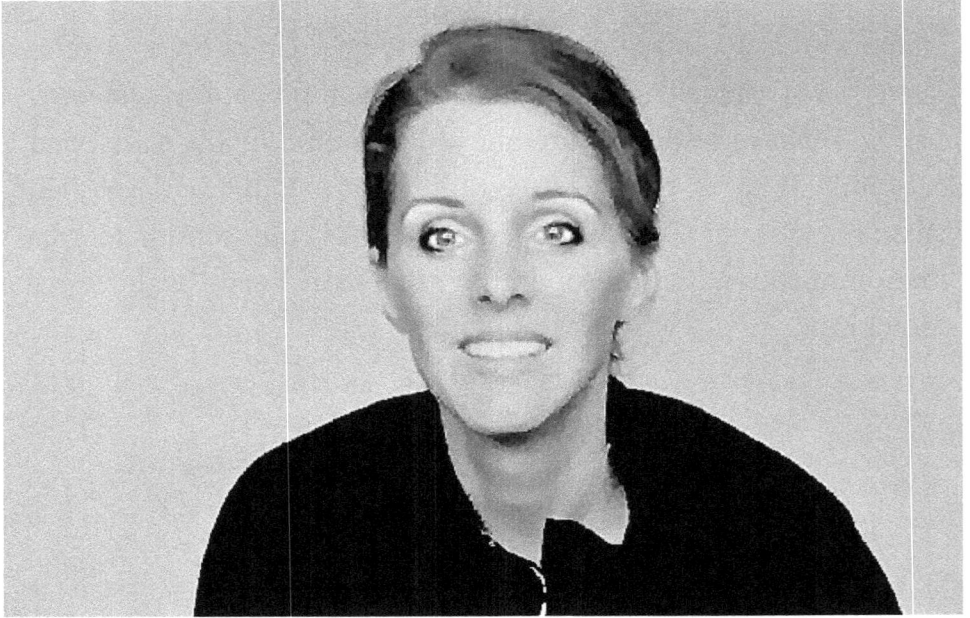

Thank you for joining us on this journey!

ABOUT THE AUTHOR

Born and raised in Michigan, growing up in a multi-season state, playing a myriad of sports throughout the year and wildly loving the adventures that changed from season to season, Dr. Cate Coker developed a love for movement, the human body and its expressive abilities in sport and recreation. She attended the University of Michigan, earning her Bachelor of Science in Biology, Bachelor of Science in Health Science and her Doctorate of Physical Therapy. Upon graduation, she was awarded the 2005 Outstanding Student Award from the Michigan Physical Therapy Association and, along with her research team, she was awarded the 2006 Student Research Award from the American Physical Therapy Association after presenting their research on a national platform in San Diego, CA. In 2015, she moved to Oahu and began a new adventure of entrepreneurship, authorship and continued work as a physical therapist there.

Her most recent project, titled "Train With Intelligence", is an endeavor to bring her unique knowledge and background into the service of athletes as they pursue excellence in their game!

REFERENCES

Coleman, D. Boyatzis, R. McKee, A. (2002). Primary
　　Leadership, Learning to Lead with Emotional
　　Intelligence. Harvard Business School Press.

Cutnell, J. Johnson, K. (1997). Physics. John Wiley &
　　Sons, Inc.

Hewitt, P. (2010). Conceptual Physics. Jim Smith.

Marieb, E. Mallat, J. (2001). Human Anatomy. Daryl Fox.

Maxwell, J. (1995). Developing the Leaders Around You, How
　　To Help Others Reach Their Potential. Injoy, Inc.

McKee, T. McKee, J. (1999). Biochemistry, An Introduction.
　　James M. Smith.

Moog, R. Farrell, J. (1999). Chemistry, A Guided Inquiry.
　　John Wiley & Sons, Inc.

Nolte, J. (1993). The Human Brain, *An Introduction to its
　　Functional Anatomy.* George Stamathis.

Silberberg, M. (2000). Chemistry, The Molecular Nature of
　　Matter and Change. James M. Smith.

Suchocki, J. (2007). Conceptual Chemistry. Jim Smith.

Thibodeau, G. Patton, K. (2004). Structure and Function of
　　the Body. Mosby.

Tortora, G. (1998). Principles of Human Anatomy. Benjamin/
　　Cummings Science Building.

www.ingramcontent.com/pod-product-compliance
Lightning Source LLC
Chambersburg PA
CBHW071845090426
42811CB00035B/2328/J